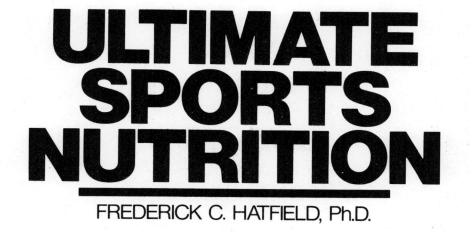

ULTIMATE SPORTS NUTRITION

FREDERICK C. HATFIELD, Ph.D.

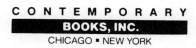

CONTEMPORARY
BOOKS, INC.
CHICAGO ▪ NEW YORK

Library of Congress Cataloging-in-Publication Data

Hatfield, Frederick C.
   Ultimate sports nutrition.

   Bibliography: p. 199
   Includes index.
   1. Athletes—Nutrition.   I. Title.   [DNLM: 1. Nutrition
—popular works.   2. Sports.   QU 145 H328u]
TX361.A8H38   1987   613.2'024796   87-8836
ISBN 0-8092-4887-5

Published by Contemporary Books, Inc.
180 North Michigan Avenue, Chicago, Illinois 60601
Manufactured in the United States of America
Library of Congress Catalog Card Number: 87-8836
International Standard Book Number: 0-8092-4887-5

Published simultaneously in Canada by Beaverbooks, Ltd.
195 Allstate Parkway, Valleywood Business Park
Markham, Ontario L3R 4T8 Canada

CONTENTS

ACKNOWLEDGMENTS

Much appreciation is given to Kelly Garrett and Linda McCrerey for their expert editing. They spent many hours helping me put very difficult subject matter into readable form.

Jerry Brainum must be given special thanks for his diligent research efforts into the often obscure and esoteric field of nutritional biochemistry. Without his help, this book most certainly would have been less than complete.

I'd also like to thank:

Dr. Michael Murray for his expert advice on amino acids;
Joe Weider and his magazine, *Sports Fitness* (for which I am editor in chief), for support and encouragement;
the hundreds of athletes out there who have aided by recounting their experiences in their quest for sports greatness.

Most of all, thanks to my family—my wife Joy, son Freddie, and daughters Disa and Kristen—for their love. They are my new beginning.

INTRODUCTION

Welcome to *Ultimate Sports Nutrition*. You, as an athlete in hard training, deserve to know about the latest advancements in nutritional science and how you can incorporate these exciting scientific breakthroughs into your own training program to help you achieve that competitive edge. And, just as important, you deserve to be able to separate fact from fiction in your quest for peak performance.

How and what to eat in foods and supplements are the subjects of this book.

If you listen to all the nonsense going around, nutrition can be a confusing subject. There are so many crackpot ideas propounded by vitamin salespeople, diet czars, self-serving quacks, and get-rich-quick hucksters that making sense out of the conflicting claims can indeed be difficult.

Unfailingly, nutrition (like certain other current topics of interest) stirs up incredibly heated debates among the know-it-alls of every imaginable extremist viewpoint. In fact, the arguments rank right up there in fever-pitch intensity with the most important issues of the day, always debated in absolute terms—the no-nuke disarmament advocates and the balance-of-terror militarists, the pro-choice advocates and the right-to-life crusaders, the feminists who protest every imaginable slight to female equality and the old guard bent on protecting the male-dominated social order.

Black or white. Good against evil. Right versus wrong. One side polarized from the other, and never the twain shall meet.

And so it is with the infant science of nutrition; many opinions are diametrically opposed. Conservative nutritionists, for example, contend that hard-training athletes don't need to supplement their diets. Pill-pushing "health" product distributors, on the other hand, insist that we athletes need megadoses of everything from bee pollen to bull's nuts.

2

Even the legitimate experts often disagree on basic scientific principles in this business. No wonder the average person has so much difficulty making his way through this informational jungle.

But we're not average people. We're athletes. And these days, everyone who exercises—even fitness-oriented nonathletes—must take the training table seriously.

We have to realize that it doesn't do us any good to take sides in the polemic battles of the extremist "experts." Nor can we afford to ignore the revolutionary scientific advancements being made in the field of sports nutrition. Our task is to tap into these breakthroughs and carefully consider how this new knowledge can be applied to our own specific training goals.

I've written *Ultimate Sports Nutrition* to show you how to do just that. Much of the information in this book is brand-new. Some has been disseminated before but bears repeating, for even athletes can be stubbornly resistant to applying basic nutritional principles. Whatever your sport, the information herein will help you achieve your true peak performance capabilities.

I suggest you read the entire book carefully once, and then clearly define your own fitness or sports goals. Reading the book first will help you crystallize in your mind just how far you will be able to take your body in your quest for sports fitness. Then, after setting your goals, decide—in writing—what to eat, when to eat it, what to take for supplements, and how you should organize your supplementation program to support your training and competition efforts.

Each step along the way will require a different supplementation approach. Off-season training goals aren't the same as preseason or in-season goals, and your nutritional support systems will have to be constantly reoriented to support the kind of training you're currently engaged in.

This is the scientific way. For serious athletes, that's the only way.

PART ONE
WE'VE COME A LONG WAY

1
WHY DO ATHLETES EAT?

Ask any typical sedentary individual why he eats, and the answer you get will be something along the lines of "To stay alive" or "Because I'm hungry." The more epicurean among those asked may add something about the pleasures of gustatory indulgence.

All well and good, but none of that has anything to do with why athletes eat. There are many reasons why athletes eat, but all of them come down to a common denominator—to win, and to excel in the process. For the athlete, the old saying "You are what you eat" takes on a new meaning in the face of the incredible leap in sophistication the science of biochemical nutrition has taken over the past few years.

The *specific* reasons that athletes consume nutrients constitute the basis of your Ultimate Sports Nutrition program. Let's look at the list:

1. To increase energy, for long-term (aerobic) and short-term (anaerobic) endurance.
2. To replace substances lost in sweat.
3. To build strength and power.
4. To build lean tissue (muscle).
5. To lose fat.

6. To enhance general health and improve functioning of all body processes.
7. To relieve pain.
8. To stimulate mental concentration.
9. To repair injuries and traumatized tissue.
10. To speed recovery between workouts.

4

Just as no one food serves all these purposes, no one athlete eats for all these reasons at any one time. As a broad example, if you are a bodybuilder whose goal is to maximize muscular size, your diet and supplements will differ from those of a triathlete who eats to increase aerobic endurance.

Your task in developing your Ultimate Sports Nutrition diet is to evaluate your goals as they pertain to the list and then apply the information in the following chapters to your reasons for eating. To know what and how to eat, you must know your specific goals. Keep those goals in mind as you absorb the latest scientific knowledge presented in the rest of this book.

The age of athletic science is upon us. It just doesn't suffice anymore to take a haphazard approach to sports training while relying merely on natural talent and instinct to achieve athletic excellence. All athletes—from fitness enthusiasts and novice competitors to "elite" athletes—can improve their performance capabilities, often dramatically, by applying state-of-the-art knowledge of training and nutrition.

Between nutrition and training, the field of nutrition presents the more complex and varied factors—and the most unknowns. But those "unknowns" are coming to light as scientific research demystifies the factors necessary for Ultimate Sports Nutrition.

Recent progress in the field of nutritional biochemistry has advanced our knowledge about what to eat, how to eat, and when to eat. We're now equipped with the biochemical wherewithal to excel beyond current standards. In an age when the winning edge is often measured in milliseconds, you, the athlete, must apply every resource to gain that edge.

Why you eat, then, is a question for which you must have adequate answers. These days, everybody who exercises or competes takes the training table seriously.

2
NUTRITIONAL NEEDS OF ATHLETES

Those of us who reside in the trenches, who compete at the highest levels of sports, are repeatedly reminded that we are not average folk. We aren't among the pigeonholed statistics hidden in an obscure computer at the Food and Drug Administration.

Indeed, what the FDA says we need to eat bears no resemblance to our true nutritional requirements. The FDA measures the *minimum* nutritional requirements for maintaining status quo health levels for sedentary people—not ultimate nutritional requirements for peak athletic performance.

If you need any further proof that an athlete's nutritional requirements are far beyond the ordinary, consider that even what passes for ordinary in this country is inadequate for minimum fitness. America, as a whole, is malnourished.

Malnutrition in the United States

It is a sad irony that in the richest nation on earth a majority of the population (60 percent) is malnourished in at least one nutrient. Despite the so-called "enrichment" of processed food in the United States, most of our citizens are not getting their *minimum* nutritional requirements. A number of recent studies substantiate this:

- The First Health and Nutrition Examination Survey in 1976 studied 28,000 persons, ages 1 to 74, in 65 areas of the United States. The study examined what they ate, the levels of certain nutrients in their blood, and symptoms of malnutrition. Findings? That 9 out of 10 females had insufficient iron in their diets, and only one-half of all females get sufficient calcium in what they eat.
- The 10-State Nutritional Survey in 1972 revealed similar nutritional deficits in the 86,000 people studied. One in three were deficient in riboflavin, a nutrient thought to be abundant in dairy products, cereals, and breads. Overall, two-thirds of the people tested showed dietary deficiencies.
- More recently, the Nationwide Food Consumption Survey in 1980 showed that one in three of the 15,000 households studied had diets deficient in calcium and pyridoxine. Deficiencies of magnesium were found in one in four diets, and iron and vitamin deficiencies were present in one in five. This is in a country known for its abundant variety and quantities of foodstuffs!

Even among people who are aware, educated, and conscientious about eating a healthy diet, about a third have nutrient deficiencies. Why? One reason that persons who make an effort to obtain adequate nutrition still come up short is that the nutrient content of foods varies widely. Worse, foods usually come nowhere near the nutrient content stated in tables published by various health agencies and hospitals. In other words, food in modern America just isn't what it's supposed to be.

For example, the amount of vitamin C in oranges varies from mere traces to 116 milligrams per 100 grams, a factor of more than 100. Fresh wheat germ can contain vitamin E in amounts ranging from 3.21 to 21 milligrams alpha-TE per 100 grams, a six-fold variation. Carrot samples, which range in quality from pale and poor to red-orange and excellent, contain from 70 micrograms beta-carotene to 1,850 micrograms per 100 grams. The RDA for betacarotene is 1,000 micrograms, so carrots eaten every day can supply either an inadequate or an excessive amount.

Minerals fare no better in food samples studies. Depending on the extent of processing, any food can vary as much as 200-fold in its mineral content. Canning, cooking, dyeing, storage, freezing, and preparation all remove minerals and vitamins from food.

The diets of average citizens (and most athletes, sad to say) are bad enough, but they're actually good compared to the scandal of nutritional deficiencies in American hospital diets. There's extensive documentation of cases of malnutrition occurring *after* patients check into a hospital, caused by the typical, devitalized hospital diet of bland, overprocessed foods.

One thing you can do to increase your chances of getting adequate nutrients from the food you eat is to seek out raw, unprocessed foods with a short transit time from grower to consumer that are grown in nutrient-rich soil. Obviously, that isn't going to provide the complete answer to the question of peak-performance nutritional requirements for athletes. For one thing, you will probably need supplements, as we will see soon.

Synergy and Biochemical Individuality

As you put together your Ultimate Sports Nutrition program based on your eating goals, your sport, and the insights in the upcoming chapters, you also have to keep in mind the variables or "problems" influencing the nutrient needs of individual athletes. The table in this chapter lists 20 of those variables, most of which are self-explanatory. A few, however, require a bit more explanation.

Synergy refers to the fact that every known nutrient may affect the action of every other. In nutrition, substances interact in multiples to produce biological functions. In other areas of science, one single substance may create one single condition. But not in nutrition. Nutrients team up, combining in different ways to cause different effects. That's synergy.

An example of nutrients that act synergistically is the interaction of vitamin D with the metabolism of calcium and phosphorus. The combined action of the B vitamins is another example, as are the interactions between vitamins E and B_{12} and vitamin E and zinc. There are even synergistic relationships between certain trace elements, such as nickel and iron, nickel and copper, copper and zinc, and calcium and magnesium.

Biochemical individuality, number two on the table, simply means that different people have different nutritional requirements. This can mean, for example, seven-fold variations in requirements for amino acids—just because each of us is different. These biochemical differences from one person to the next form what Michael Colgan, Ph.D., director of the Colgan Institute of Nutritional Science, calls "the tip of the genetic iceberg . . . most of which remains to be investigated."

Biochemical individuality applies to more than just genetic differences, though. It can also be rooted in environmental sources, such as temperature, heavy sweating, intensity of exercise, and other stressors that increase nutrient needs. Athletes as a whole are in a different biochemical condition than the average person because they expose themselves to more of these stressors more often. And, of course, biochemical individuality varies from athlete to athlete.

8

A final item in the table that needs some explanation is *physiological dynamics*, which has to do with the time it takes for a supplementation program to take effect. We'll talk about that in Chapter 9.

The bottom line is that we athletes need a higher level of nutrition than the average sedentary person. We know this because over the years we've been tuning into our bodies' needs. And finally, what we know from experience is receiving scientific support from nutritional biochemists and exercise physiologists.

Until recently, most conventional nutritionists have missed the boat with athletes. Perhaps they've been too preoccupied by taking care of bed-ridden invalids or elderly folks or doing surveys to justify governmental cutbacks in food stamps. They hadn't been paying attention to the leading edge in human performance—the athlete.

Our list of why athletes eat—your guide to formulating your Ultimate Sports Nutrition program—may be incomplete. There are certainly overlapping factors regarding how athletes metabolize nutrients. And not every item on the list is going to apply to you as an individual athlete. But experience tells us that none of these functions can be achieved through normal eating patterns.

At least not if you aspire to athletic greatness.

Variables Influencing Nutrient Needs of Individual Athletes

1. Synergy. Nutrients operate by multiple interactions
2. Biochemical Individuality
3. Race
4. Family Medical History
5. Individual Medical History
6. Current Medication
7. Lifestyle and Environment
8. Living and working environment
9. Exercise
10. Individual Diet
11. Bioavailability of Nutrients
12. Current nutritional status
13. Air and Water Pollution
14. Food Pollution
15. Food Degradation
16. Food Processing
17. Food Additive Combinations
18. Food Storage and Preparation
19. Excretion of Nutrients
20. Physiological Dynamics

PART TWO
THE BIOCHEMISTRY OF
ENHANCED PERFORMANCE

3
PROTEIN

How much protein do you, the serious athlete, need to consume for peak performance capability? That question is a keystone to constructing your Ultimate Sports Nutrition program. Not surprisingly, it's a controversial subject.

Reading the latest relevant scientific literature on protein requirements is bound to confuse you totally. Recommendations at each extreme of the scale differ by as much as 100 percent! Depending on which expert conducted the study, you're supposed to eat anywhere from 0.925 grams to 2.0 grams of protein per kilogram of body weight per day. In pounds of body weight, that translates to .42 to 1.0 grams of protein per pound per day, more than a 100-percent difference between the two numbers.

To sort through the maze and get at a daily intake that makes sense for you, you need to look at your special needs as an athlete and the nature of protein itself.

The RDA Factor

The first thing you do is forget about the "Recommended Daily Allowances" (RDAs) set by the National Research Council. Even among the widely varying opinions of sports scientists and nutritionists, that's a point of agreement. The RDAs are far too low even for fitness buffs who exercise regularly, let alone for serious athletes interested in peak performance.

The National Research Council's RDA for protein consumption is 0.42 grams per day per pound of body weight (or 0.93 grams per kilogram). That means that an athlete weighing 120 pounds requires 50 grams of protein per day.

This, of course, is hogwash. If you follow what the National Research Council says, you'll turn into a mullet, an average pencil-necked slob who doesn't work out. The typical male mullet carries about 20 percent body fat and leads a sedentary life. So forget the RDA for protein. It has nothing to do with you.

Why You Need Protein

Protein is a builder. Unlike carbohydrates, which function primarily as a ready-made fuel source for the body, protein's role is to form building material.

There's more protein in your body than any other substance except for water. It's present in virtually every organ in your body, and it's required for the growth and development of all body tissues. Blood, muscles, the heart, the brain, skin, hair, and nails—these are all formed primarily of protein. Good health and vitality depend on protein.

You also need protein to produce hormones, which regulate a host of body functions, including growth, metabolic rate, and sexual development. Protein regulates the acid-alkaline balance in your blood and maintains proper water balance in your body. It's necessary for the formation of enzymes, which are required for basic life functions. It helps form antibodies, basic components of your immune system. It's needed in everything from the production of mother's milk to the process of blood clotting.

Protein deficiency can result in growth abnormalities and impaired tissue development. Your hair, nails, and skin will suffer, and your muscle will lose its tone. While protein deficiency can stunt the growth of children, it's manifested in adults as tiredness and low energy, mental depression, weakness, low resistance to infection (because of an impaired immune system), slow healing of wounds, and slow recovery from disease.

Eating too much protein has the same result as eating too much fat or carbohydrates: your liver will convert it into fat, and it will be stored in the body tissues. Protein, however, has about half the concentration of calories contained in any fat you may consume. A gram of protein contains about 5.65 calories, roughly equivalent to carbohydrates (4.1) in energy value.

Protein and Your Diet

When you digest protein, the molecules are broken down into *amino acids*, smaller units often called "the building blocks of protein." To make human protein, 22 amino acids, constructed in a certain pattern, are required. But your body produces only 12 of those in sufficient quantities.

The other ten are called *essential amino acids*, and they *must be obtained from your diet*. If even one essential amino acid is low or missing from your diet, synthesis of all the other amino acids will be reduced to the same level as the deficient or absent one. As you can see, protein synthesis is complex and delicate, and that fact is reflected in the protein efficiency ratio (PER) of the foods you eat.

That's why, using PER as a guide, you should pay attention to the *quality* of protein you consume in your diet. You have to make sure that the whole complement of amino acids is supplied. So-called protein foods vary in the numbers and proportions of the amino acids they contain. For example, most meats and dairy products are considered "complete" protein foods because they contain all ten essential amino acids. Most vegetables and fruits, on the other hand, are considered "incomplete" protein foods. Keep in mind, though, that it's possible to supply complete proteins in a meal made up of incomplete protein foods by carefully combining menu items.

Another factor of protein nourishment represented in the protein efficiency ratio is *assimilation*. That simply refers to the amount of consumed protein that is actually digested, absorbed, and metabolized by your body. Eggs, for example, top the list of amounts of usable protein—a 96 percent PER—because they contain all ten essential amino acids in the proper proportion. In fact, eggs are the standard by which all other protein sources are rated in terms of assimilability. Milk is second highest, with about a 60 percent PER. Next are the meats, ranging near 40 percent PER. Vegetables rate 15 percent PER at best.

A good rule of thumb is to eat even more protein than the eventual daily intake figure you come up with, because part of what you consume will be wasted protein. In other words, it will be incomplete protein that won't be assimilated. Also, you can maximize your protein assimilation by including both meat and milk in your diet and by taking amino acid supplements.

Protein and the Athlete

One of the reasons that the RDA is useless for you is that it indicates only the basic protein level required to maintain health under usual environmental stress. The actual dietary protein requirement depends on several variable factors—including age, individual nutritional status, body size, and activity level.

Also, protein is depleted from the body during periods of physical stress—such as surgery, hemorrhage, injuries, prolonged illness, and heavy training. When you're stressed or training extra hard, therefore, you should consume more protein to bolster the healing and developmental processes of your body and to rebuild and replace damaged tissues.

As an athlete, you incur additional protein losses through heavy sweating, blood cell destruction, major injuries, repeated minor injuries (such as strains, sprains, and inflammation), and the ongoing physiological stress of heavy exercise.

If you lift weights to build muscle, you have an even higher protein requirement for muscle growth. During those periods when you may be dieting to reduce body fat, your protein requirement increases.

Clearly, your status as an athlete engaging in frequent heavy exercise has a profound effect on your protein intake requirement. But why exactly does the stress of heavy exercise mean that your body needs more protein? The answer has to do with the mechanics of protein metabolism.

Protein production and protein breakdown—the two aspects of the ongoing process of protein metabolism—exist in a dynamic balance, resulting in the maintenance of a constant body weight. Muscle is the major depot of protein in the body, and a significant increase or decrease in the mass of body protein is likely to affect muscle protein in particular, changing muscle weight and strength accordingly.

Exercise promotes a *decrease* in protein production that continues for several hours *after* exercise. Over time, this would result in a major loss of muscle mass and weight if it weren't for the period of increased production that follows the period of decreased production of protein. That's why it's so important to allow sufficient recovery time between exercise bouts. Allowing insufficient recovery time for this period of increased protein production may be the underlying cause of impaired athletic performance from overtraining.

Why does exercise cause accelerated protein breakdown? There are two theories. One has to do with the use of protein as a fuel source for muscle contraction. It may seem counterproductive for a muscle to derive energy from its own tissues, but that's exactly what it does; muscle has the ability to use protein for energy and does so while in the resting state. Consequently, large stores of energy are present in the body in this form. The quantity of protein used as an exercise fuel seems to increase during prolonged aerobic exercise such as long-distance running, swimming, and cycling.

Another theory about exercise causing protein breakdown is related to amino acids. Since they're the building blocks of protein, maintaining an adequate supply of amino acids ensures maximal rates of protein production. Growth depends on adequate quantities of amino acids through protein consumption. Since regular weight training increases muscle growth (hypertrophy), the need for protein is elevated.

Finding the Protein Allowance for You

You must consider all the variables when you design the appropriate protein allowance for your particular sport—and your particular body.

Endurance athletes, take note! Biochemical studies conducted in the last few years suggest that the protein metabolism during endurance exercise is much higher than previously thought. It's now estimated that protein provides 5 to 15 percent of the energy for endurance exercise. That means that endurance athletes need to consume an increased amount of protein.

Elite-level athletes who are well supported nutritionally and otherwise for endurance exercise can use as an appropriate figure for protein requirement 1.5–2.0 grams per kilogram of body weight, or about .7–1.0 grams per pound. Note that this is nearly *double the amount recommended by the FDA* for the average person under usual conditions. This amount maintains positive nitrogen balance over weeks of heavy training.

Using these figures as a base, you can calculate your individual protein requirement for your own weight. For example, if you're a 110-pound athlete, you need 75–110 grams of first-class (i.e., complete) protein daily. If you weigh 154 pounds, you need 105–154 grams. If you're 220 pounds, you require 150–220 grams.

If your protein consumption dips below this level—if you're trying to avoid the fats in meat and dairy products, for example—you'd better take amino acid or protein supplements to maintain adequate protein levels.

Another way to figure your protein requirements, good for strength and endurance athletes, is by percentage. Marathon runners and triathletes require 10 to 12 percent of their daily diet from complete proteins. Strength athletes such as football linemen and powerlifters need 15 to 20 percent.

Remember: not all protein in the food you eat is totally assimilated because of imbalances in the essential amino acids. Therefore, you should eat more protein foods than you need, knowing that part of the total will be wasted.

As you can see, your Ultimate Sports Nutrition eating plan calls for more protein than you may have thought. Weightlifters and other strength athletes do need slightly more protein than endurance athletes, but not nearly as much as previously believed. This does not mean, however, that all limits on protein are off. Stuffing yourself with a dozen eggs a day plus two steaks and a quart of milk may add size, but it won't be the muscular kind. It will be fat—

Protein and Caloric Requirements as Recommended by Various Countries for Different Age Groups

	Age	Weight (kilos)	Calories	Protein (grams)	Percent of Calories as Protein
USA	15–18	66	2,600	56	6.2
	19–22	70	2,900	56	7.9
	23–50	70	2,700	56	8.5
Canada	16–18	64	3,200	54	6.9
	19–35	70	3,000	56	7.6
	36–50	70	2,700	56	8.5
Britain	15–18	56	2,300	68	12.1
	18–35	65	3,000	75	10.2
	35–65	65	2,900	73	10.3
Japan	18	61	2,650	80	12.4
	30	63	2,400	70	11.9
	50	59	2,200	70	13.0
Russia	14–17	—	2,700	93	13.8
	18–40	—	3,000	99	13.5
	40–60	—	2,800	92	13.4

Note: Observe the substantial difference between Russia and the other countries with regard to recommended protein allowances. Note too that by simple interpolation procedures, one can get a fairly close estimate of one's protein requirements for any body weight. However, it's best to calculate your caloric needs first, and then multiply that by the percentage recommended in this book for protein allowances (10–20 percent of your daily calories—lower for endurance athletes, higher for power athletes and bodybuilders).

layering the body and clogging the arteries. There are better ways to die than from heart disease and obesity.

Overconsumption of protein causes another undesirable effect: formation of a highly toxic ammonia called *urea*. Urea must be excreted from the system, and that places a strain on the liver and kidneys. If you're a weightlifter who uses anabolic steroids, those organs already are severely impacted.

15

4
CARBOHYDRATES

For you as an athlete, the most important feature of carbohydrates is that they yield *instantly available* calories to give you energy for both aerobic and anaerobic activities. Your Ultimate Sports Nutrition program should contain a high percentage of carbohydrates: from 50 to 60 percent for strength athletes and from 70 to 80 percent for endurance athletes.

The different physiological requirements for different types of sports dictate the relative demands for carbohydrates and proteins. Start paying attention to your carbohydrate consumption. Get to know the differences among the types of carbohydrates and how your body uses them. This information will help you design your Ultimate Sports Nutrition diet.

What Are Carbohydrates?

Carbohydrates—consisting chemically of various combinations of carbon, hydrogen, and oxygen molecules—come in three categories:

- *Simple sugars* (glucose, fructose, and galactose), such as those found in honey and fruits, are known scientifically as *monosaccharides.*

- *Sucrose*, or table sugar, comes under the heading of *disaccharides*. (Lactose and maltose are also disaccharides.)
- *Complex carbohydrates*, the starches (dextrins, cellulose, pectin, and glycogen) such as those found in whole grains and legumes, are *polysaccharides*.

18

One important component of carbohydrates, cellulose, is found in the skins of fruits and vegetables. Humans cannot digest cellulose, so it's useless for energy. But it provides fiber necessary for normal digestion and regular elimination of wastes.

The best way to understand the composition of carbohydrates is to look at a single kernel of corn. The outer layer of the kernel contains the 12 percent of this food source that's indigestible—the cellulose, hemicellulose, and lignin that make up the roughage that passes through your system and is excreted in the feces. This has its uses, including protecting your digestive tract from disorders, promoting regularity, and discouraging overeating by creating a full feeling.

Inside, the kernel is composed of simple sugars and sucrose (these two categories are usually lumped together as *simple carbohydrates* for convenience) and of complex starches. Thus, corn is a relatively complete source of carbohydrates, with the digestible portion providing vitamins and minerals the way nature intended: together. The simple carbohydrates in corn and other whole grains enhance flavor but are prevented from entering the bloodstream too quickly.

Carbs for Energy

How important are carbohydrates to your performance? *Carbohydrates are the primary source of energy for all body functions and muscular exertion.* Your digestive system converts all sugars and starches to glucose, or "blood sugar." Your muscle cells are able to store a small quantity of fuel—glucose is converted to muscle glycogen for storage inside the muscle cells—but the immediate energy needs of your brain and working muscles are supplied by this blood-borne glucose.

If there is blood glucose left over (and there will be if you've overeaten), after a period of two or three hours after eating, the excess is converted to adipose tissue—stored energy.

The key to manipulating your carbohydrate intake for optimal athletic performance is to know the rates at which carbohydrates are converted to blood sugar and metabolized as energy. The most important thing to remember is this: the complex carbohydrates found in whole grains, nuts, vegetables, and some fruits become blood sugar at a slow rate, yielding energy for exercise over a prolonged period at a stable rate. That's why complex carbohydrates are the preferred fuel for athletic activities.

Carbohydrate foods such as peas, grains, corn, and pasta are popular menu items at pre-event meals because their complex molecular structures provide long-term energy. These meals can at times take the form of "carbohydrate loading," which we'll talk about later in the book (see Chapter 30). The main point here is that you need lots of carbohydrates to get the glucose and glycogen you need as the primary ingredients in fuel for exercise. (Before you get carried away, though, remember that carbohydrates aren't *all* you need; proper amounts of fat and protein are important as well.)

Because muscular exertion in endurance events is limited by the amount of glycogen stored in your muscles, you'll experience a sudden and extreme fatigue when the stores are depleted. Marathon runners call this "hitting the wall," and long-distance cyclists refer to it as "bonking." That's why carbo loading can be a valuable tool in the aresenal of Ultimate Sports Nutrition techniques. By increasing your available muscle glycogen, you'll be able to carry on with the race instead of slowing down drastically or dropping out. It's a classic illustration of what nutrition can do for an athlete that all the training in the world can't.

Here's one final illustration of the important fact that complex carbohydrates yield a greater supply of muscle glycogen (your fuel) than simple carbohydrates do. A recent study (Costill) involved feeding male runners a diet of either 70 percent complex carbohydrates or 70 percent simple carbohydrates 48 hours after a run that had depleted their glycogen reserves. Result: 20 percent greater glycogen repletion for the complex carb group.

The Sins of Sugar

Sugar is an insidious bandit of sound nutrition. It's also addictive. All you have to do is compare the effects of eating energy-producing complex carbohydrates with the effects of consuming simple carbohydrates—table sugar, milk lactose, and maltose—and you should be convinced. The former are a superior source of energy for athletes; the latter lead to trouble.

Simple carbohydrates are really a form of "predigested" sugar:

they become blood glucose very rapidly. That's why snacks and meals high in sugar or processed white flour or polished rice will give you an initial rush of energy. Your blood sugar is soaring. The subsequent sudden letdown as your blood sugar level plummets leads to muscle fatigue, dizziness, nervousness, and headaches—and a craving for another fix of sugar. Needless to say, none of this does your athletic performance any good.

20

People who eat too much sugar and processed grains in place of other essential foods usually suffer from nutritional deficiencies, as well as obesity and tooth decay. Simple carbohydrates are typically low in vitamins, minerals, and cellulose. Overconsumption of sugar inhibits carbohydrate metabolism, so it shouldn't be a surprise that a sweet tooth pigout is usually accompanied by indigestion, heartburn, and nausea.

If you eat a lot of sugar, you're flirting with hypertension, heart disease, diabetes. Further, there are links between sugar consumption and criminal tendencies. Even cancer is a possible consequence.

Michael Colgan, Ph.D., one of the nation's premier sports nutritionists, makes a case against sugar that is of special interest to athletes. Colgan maintains that the sudden rise and fall of blood sugar created by pre-exercise snacks of sugar actually accelerate the loss of muscle glycogen. That means reduced performance.

Want more evidence? Simple carbohydrate consumption increases your uric acid levels, reduces glucose tolerance, impairs lipid metabolism, and elevates levels of cholesterols and triglycerides.

Even the Food and Drug Administration, which you may have gathered by now is usually a conservative organization, recently issued a statement to the effect that if it had known 50 years ago what it knows now, sugar would have been banned from the grocery shelves as a deadly poison!

So don't shrug off your sugar binges as a harmless habit. Wise up, fellow athletes, and shun the simple carbohydrates in favor of what your body really needs: *complex* carbohydrates.

Use the Glycemic Index

Separating the good from the bad carbohydrates is more complex than simple, so to speak. In fact, it can get a little tricky. That's because not all simple carbohydrates have the same yo-yo effect on your blood glucose. And not all complex carbohydrates take a long time to break down into blood sugar.

So how do you pick and choose? Science has done the work for you by charting various carbohydrate foods on a Glycemic Index (see the accompanying table), based on blood glucose response. For example, apples and oranges have relatively slow burning rates, making these foods desirable fuel sources for athletes. Whole wheat, oats, and brown rice are other good athletic energy choices from the carbohydrates category.

The Glycemic Index of Various Foods

EAT LESS OF THESE		EAT MORE OF THESE	
Food	**Glycemic Index**	**Food**	**Glycemic Index**
Sugars		*Sugars*	
Glucose	100	Fructose	20
Honey	87		
Vegetables		*Vegetables*	
Parsnips	98	Soybeans	15
Carrots	90	Kidney beans	30
White potatoes	70	Lentils	25
		Sweet potatoes	48
Fruit		*Fruit*	
Bananas	65	Apples	36
Raisins	68	Oranges	40
Dates	72		
Grains		*Grains*	
White flour spaghetti	56	Whole wheat spaghetti	40
Cornflakes	85	Oats	48
White rice	70	Brown rice	60
White flour pancakes	66	Buckwheat pancakes	45
White bread	76	Whole wheat bread	64

The Glycemic Index may contain some surprises for you. Carrots, white potatoes, bananas, and white rice have high glycemic values and cause a rapid rise and fall of blood sugar levels. You may have thought of these as healthful foods, but they should be on the athlete's "eat less" list for pregame energy.

A word about fructose. This fruit sugar, available in health food stores in white powder form, does indeed have a low Glycemic Index of 20, meaning that it is metabolized by the system at a relatively slow rate. At first glance you would think fructose is the ideal athletic energy food. After all, it has little effect on your blood glucose level, and it significantly spares muscle glycogen stores when you ingest it just prior to exercise. And it is indeed on the "eat more" side of the chart.

But Dr. Colgan advises against the overindulgence of all forms of sugar—fructose included—because of the impact sugar has on increased triglyceride production. Triglycerides are implicated in coronary heart diseases when their levels remain high over prolonged periods.

However, athletes in hard training apparently need not fear coronary damage stemming from elevated blood triglycerides, since most have far lower levels than the average sedentary person.

In any event, it's probably advisable to stick to fresh fruits instead of the powder form for your fructose intake.

An Object Lesson for Athletes

There's one group of athletes that need to be especially reminded of the importance of complex carbohydrates: competitive bodybuilders. Bodybuilders, who are often looked to as the standard for all strength athletes, traditionally reduce drastically or eliminate carbohydrates from their diets three or four weeks before a competition. This practice needs to be addressed, because it can lead an athlete down the road to trouble.

The theory is that, in order to get as lean, cut, and defined as possible, a bodybuilder should shun carbohydrates as a competition nears because they cause retention of water in the system (anathema to bodybuilders) and add unwanted calories. Instead, a high-protein diet supposedly is necessary in the weeks before the contest.

While carbohydrates do retain water, they don't do so to such an extent to warrant their exclusion from the diet for any extended period. And while it's also true that a high-protein diet can help in losing weight, it is *not* true that complex carbs make you fat. In fact, they contain roughage and fiber that enhance the digestive process, and their calories are readily burned.

So forget bodybuilding tradition. Complex carbohydrates should be included in any athlete's diet because a total lack of them produces ketosis (energy loss, depression, and a breakdown of essential body protein) and ultimately, death. In fact, anybody who's been around the bodybuilding scene knows that most competitors get unbearably irritable and depressed as the contest approaches. That's because they've been denying their body carbohydrates. You actually can start feeling ill and depressed after just three days of carbohydrate deprivation.

So instead of feeling on top of the world—healthy, strong, vibrant, in the best shape of your life, a winner—you feel hopeless, jittery, weak, and wasted, and you wonder if it's all worth it. That's no way for an athlete to feel. In addition, you'll have bad breath from ketosis and constipation from dietary fiber deficiency.

You don't need a doctorate in biochemistry to realize by now that the bodybuilder's traditional no-carbohydrate precontest diet is unhealthful and counterproductive. Bodybuilders should replace it with a more sensible diet that is perhaps lower in calories and fat than usual but that contains adequate complex carbohydrates and protein.

All athletes need to make wise decisions about carbohydrates as they relate to their Ultimate Sports Nutrition program. To help you in the task, refer to the accompanying tables, which list the best grains and legumes for high complex carbohydrate, high protein, low fat, and sufficient fiber content. Bear in mind that, even if you're an endurance athlete striving for as much as 80 percent complex carbohydrates in your diet, the actual level consumed might be closer to 68 percent because of the amount of nutrient-destroying processing that goes into the foods in a typical American diet.

Top 20 Grains and Legumes for Athletes

Best Protein Sources **Over 20% Protein** **Under 20% Fat**	Best Carbohydrate Sources **Under 5% Fat** **Over 70% Carbohydrate**
Soybeans	Brown Rice
Split Peas	Whole Barley
Kidney Beans	Whole Buckwheat
Dried Whole Peas	Whole Rye
Wheat Germ	Foxtail Millet
Lima Beans	Wild Rice
Black-Eyed Peas	Whole Corn
Lentils	Pearl Millet
Black Beans	Whole Wheat
Navy Beans	Rolled Oats

Fiber "10"
(Each contains 10 grams of dietary fiber.)

Grains	Vegetables	Fruits
½ cup All Bran	½ cup Mixed Beans	3 Pears
1 cup Rolled Oats	½ cup Peas, Lentils	3 Bananas
1 cup Whole Grain Cereal	1 cup Peanuts	4 Peaches
2 cobs Sweet Corn	2 cups Soybeans	4 oz. Blackberries
3 slices Whole Rye Bread	3 cups Steamed Vegetables	5 Apples
3 cups Puffed Wheat	4 servings Mixed Salad	6 Oranges
4 slices Whole Wheat Bread	4 large Carrots	6 Dried Pear Halves
4 Shredded Wheat	4 cups Sunflower Seeds	10 Dried Figs
4-oz. bag Popcorn	5 cups raw Cauliflower	20 Prunes

5
FATS

To athletes, fats should be thought of as a secondary source of energy during physical exercise. That's exactly what they are. Fats are called into play after readily available muscle glycogen stores are depleted. That depletion occurs after about 30 to 45 minutes of vigorous aerobic exercise performed at about 70 to 75 percent of your maximum heart rate.

So forget about the popular notion that fats are nothing but bad for your body. The truth is that some fat intake is necessary for normal body functions.

Also known as *lipids*, fats provide you with the most concentrated source of energy, more than double the caloric value of protein or carbohydrates. Those concentrated calories in fat are as much a danger as a bonus, though, so beware. Not all fats are alike, and a basic understanding of their characteristics is essential to your Ultimate Sports Nutrition program for peak performance.

The Functions of Fat

The energy that fats provide is only one of their vital functions. Here are some of the reasons why you need fats in your diet:

- Fats carry vitamins A, D, E, and K, known as the *fat-soluble vitamins*. In fact, without the presence of adequate fats, your

body cannot absorb vitamin D and carry calcium to your bones and teeth. You also need fats to convert carotene to vitamin A.
- Fats cushion and protect your vital organs, including your kidneys, heart, nerve tissues, and liver.
- Subcutaneous fat—the fat under your skin—insulates your body from heat loss.
- That satisfied feeling of fullness after eating is provided by fats, which slow the digestive process by inhibiting secretions of hydrochloric acid in your stomach.
- It's fats, via fatty acids, that give your foods flavor and texture. The fact is, if you eliminate all fats from your diet, you're likely to feel deprived and depressed. Those feelings come more from the lack of flavors and hence esthetic enjoyment of eating than from the calories eliminated.

So everybody needs a certain amount of dietary fat, including athletes. The trick is to consume the right kinds in the right amounts.

Fatty Acids

Those fats that are nutritionally desirable are composed of three essential unsaturated "fatty acids": linoleic, arachidonic, and linolenic acids. The key word here is *unsaturated*. These are the ones that are necessary for normal growth, as well as healthy blood, arteries, and nerves. If you don't get these essential fatty acids, you're risking flakiness and dryness of skin and scalp and eczema. It's also these essential unsaturated fatty acids that help transport and break down cholesterol.

The other kind of fatty acid is *saturated*. The saturated fatty acids are derived mainly from animal sources, and they harden at room temperature. Well-known examples include butter, lard, tallow, and blubber. *Avoid saturated fats.* They metabolize slowly, clog the arteries, and contribute to heart disease.

Here's something to keep in mind: coconut oil is obviously not an animal fat, but it falls under the saturated fat category. Unfortunately, coconut oil is a common ingredient in store-bought cookies, crackers, and baked goods. So your elimination of saturated fats from your diet is going to require some careful reading of the labels on packaged foods.

Unsaturated fatty acids—the kind you want—come primarily from vegetable, nut, and seed sources. They stay liquid at room temperature. Common household cooking and salad oils made from corn, safflower, sunflowers, soy, and olives are unsaturated fats. An excellent nonvegetable source of unsaturated fats is cod-liver oil.

There are subcategories of unsaturated fats that you've probably heard of: polyunsaturated (including safflower, sunflower, and corn oils) and monounsaturated (peanut, olive, and avocado oils). You used to hear nutritionists recommending that you consume only the polyunsaturates, in the mistaken belief that monounsaturates were linked to heart disease. But the newest research indicates that both are needed for good health, and it's an imbalance that may actually contribute to heart disease.

So don't be afraid to pass up the blue cheese salad dressing and grab the olive oil instead. Avoid the saturated fats, and keep a balance between your intake of polyunsaturated and your consumption of monounsaturated fats.

Dietary Fats and Body Fat

So now let's get to the question that's no doubt been on your mind throughout this discussion: How much of my diet should be fats, and how can I make sure I get what I need without gaining unwanted weight?

The bad rap about fats comes from the ease with which fat deposits seem to grow on our bodies. But the fact is that any type of calories—fat, protein, or carbohydrates—can turn to fat if we ingest more than we burn. Fats are by no means the only culprit in obesity. The real culprit is a haphazard diet that doesn't consider balance or the lifestyle of the eater.

Still, the average American consumes fats at the whopping rate of 45 percent of his daily diet. That amount becomes even more staggering when you consider that it's as much as 400 percent of his actual nutritional requirement.

Fats should make up 10 to 15 percent of your total calories. This is seemingly a nearly impossible task to the average American, who has a hard time keeping his fat consumption to a limit of 23 percent. But it is because of overconsumption of fats that Americans suffer so much indigestion, obesity, and heart disease.

Even though an athlete's lifestyle is obviously more active than that of the average American, athletes, too, should stick to 10 to 15 percent fats. You already know that your primary source of long-term energy is carbohydrates. You do need fats for the reasons we've discussed—secondary energy and other bodily functions. However, fat deficiency is almost unheard of in humans because so many common foods contain fats—especially milk (except skim milk), cheese, eggs, nuts, seeds, and meat. So your task is to limit your fat intake, to avoid saturated fats, and to strike a balance between polyunsaturated and monounsaturated fats.

It's also recommended that the essential fatty acid linoleic acid, found in vegetable oils, provide about 2 percent of your total calories. To accomplish that, consume most of your dietary fats from light vegetable oils, fish, nuts, and seeds. Be sparing in your consumption of dairy products such as butter, cheese, and eggs. Animal flesh is marbled with saturated fat and should be eaten even more sparingly.

A final word of caution to you athletes who work out mainly with weights. Strength athletes rarely venture into the high-calorie-burning aerobic pathway for energy as do endurance athletes. So the 10–15 percent limitation is especially important. You don't burn enough calories to be careless with your fat intake.

With fats, a little goes a long way.

6
CALORIES

Food energy comes from three things: carbohydrates, protein, and fats. Calories are simply a way of measuring the energy those nutrients provide. As an athlete, your interest in calories focuses on the maintenance of an ideal body weight. You simply must design into your Ultimate Sports Nutrition program a calorie intake that equals calorie output.

More precisely, calories measure that amount of chemical energy that is released as heat when food is metabolized. One calorie equals the amount of heat required to raise the temperature of one gram of water one degree centigrade.

Conveniently, the caloric content (that is, the fuel potential) can be measured for the three different food types. Carbohydrates and proteins yield about four calories per gram, and fats yield about nine calories per gram.

For all that's been written about them, there's really no mystique about how calories work. Your food intake is converted to glycogen and stored in your muscles for burning during activity. The excess is stored in the body in the form of fat. Get a handle on how many calories you burn, adjust your calorie consumption accordingly, and you've mastered weight control. It's that simple.

Your body is never doing nothing. Even when you're inactive, your body requires energy to repair and maintain cells, build muscle, and carry on basic body functions, like breathing and digestion. So the total number of calories you would use over a 24-hour period while lying quietly in bed (not asleep, but awake and quiet) is a useful measurement against which you can compare yourself with other individuals as well as against different levels of activity on any given day. It's called your basal metabolic rate, or BMR.

Age, sex, body size, body weight, and endocrine function are some of the variables influencing BMR. Still, we can generalize that the average 20-year-old man has a BMR of one calorie per hour for each kilogram (2.2046 pounds) of body weight for each 24-hour period. (For a woman of the same age, it's about 0.9 calories).

So we can use that formula to figure an approximate daily expenditure of calories. For example, a 154-pound man burns about 70 calories per hour sleeping, or 560 calories in an eight-hour period. The same man burns about 80 calories an hour lying quietly awake. Normal light daily activities—walking around, studying, working at a desk—burn about 100 calories an hour if you weigh 154 pounds.

If you know what you generally do all day, you can compute your energy requirements by using the energy costs table presented here. Remember, these calorie counts are for a 154-pound man. You can adjust for differences in body weight by adding or subtracting 10 calories per hour per activity for each five pounds' difference from our hypothetical case. But even then, the table provides only an *estimate*, because, as mentioned before, BMRs vary due to a number of factors.

You can elevate your BMR by manipulating your exercise program. New knowledge confirms that people who exercise aerobically for 30 to 45 minutes at 75 percent of capacity *continue to burn calories at an escalated rate for several hours after exercising.* Also, after a few weeks of training, your BMR will increase. What all this no doubt means is that, as an athlete, you have a resting metabolism that is higher than that of the average sedentary person, allowing you to burn more calories throughout the day.

Calories, then, are important to your Ultimate Sports Nutrition program. You need to become aware of the basic caloric requirements of your activities so you can adjust your caloric intake accordingly. This is especially important when your goal is gaining or losing weight, but it also matters for everyday body weight maintenance.

Energy Costs of Various Activities

Physical Activity	Estimated Kcal/hour	Physical Activity	Estimated Kcal/hour
Archery	270	Running (7-minute mile)	950
Badminton	400	Singing	120
Basketball	560	Sitting in Class	90
Billiards	235	Skating	470
Bowling	215	Skiing (Nordic)	1,080
Bull Session	90	Skipping Rope	800
Calisthenics	200	Sleeping	70
Cleaning	185	Soccer	540
Cooking	240	Softball	280
Cycling (5 mph)	300	Squash	650
Disco	450	Studying/Reading	105
Dressing	200	Swimming	500
Driving to class	180	Table Tennis	280
Field Hockey	560	Television	90
Gardening	295	Tennis	450
Golf	340	Volleyball	255
Gymnastics	257	Walking to Class	300
Jogging	750	Walking up Stairs	180
Lying Quietly	80	Washing and Shaving	150
Marathon Running	990	Weight Training	550
Playing Cards	140	Wood Chopping	560
Racquet Sports	870	Wrestling	790
Rowing (6 mph)	900		

7
VITAMINS AND MINERALS

Here it is, the eve of the 21st century, and most of us still have primitive notions of the importance of vitamins and minerals. Don't feel bad; you're in good company. The precise mechanisms by which many minerals work remain unclear even to biochemists, and nutritionists still bicker among themselves over the quantities, the balance, and even the need for dietary supplements. Some people still maintain that the mythical "balanced diet" will supply everything you need, but the truth is that the American trend is toward progressively less nutritious, more processed food.

The fact remains that, because you're an athlete, you use up more vitamins and minerals. You want to get the most out of your body, and to do that you must supply it with everything it needs. Sports science is helping you toward that end by defining some of the specific physiological benefits those individual vitamins and minerals have.

Your unique experience is important here, though. Two athletes can be the same weight and size, play the same sport, and eat the same foods, yet they might require completely different dietary supplements. Although there's no substitute for professional nutritional guidance, you can do a lot for your body armed only with this book and a careful inventory of your dietary habits and physical sensations. And bear in mind that the effects of supplements are usually subtle and show themselves only over time—don't expect a vitamin packet to take two minutes off your mile time, at least not on the first day.

Vitamins

Vitamin A

34

Protein enables cells to build and repair themselves, and vitamin A enables your body to make and absorb protein. Working its magic in the liver, A is essential to the process of stringing together digested amino acids to form longer protein molecules. If there's insufficient A in your system, your body can't heal itself, and everything from skin to organs to bones suffers.

The vitamin comes in two forms, carotene and retinol. Green, yellow, and orange vegetables and fruits, such as spinach, cantaloupe, carrots, beans, and yams, are prime sources of carotene. Your body converts carotene into retinol, which is found ready-made in eggs, fish-liver oils, and organ meats.

If your diet consists largely of fast foods, overcooked vegetables, and red meat, there's a good chance you're missing out on vitamin A. Deficiency isn't rare—in the states of Texas and Washington, for example, one-third of the women and one-quarter of the men were found to lack sufficient vitamin A. Early symptoms of deficiency include night blindness, hardening and roughening of the skin, and degeneration of mucous membrances. You should incorporate as many fresh and raw vegetables into your diet as possible, but be aware that researchers have found that one carrot can have 26 times as much beta-carotene as another, as stated earlier. Unless you analyze your food chemically before you eat it, the only trustworthy sources of vitamin A are dietary supplements.

B Complex Vitamins

Originally thought to be a single substance, the Bs are actually a number of organic chemicals that depend on and complement one another. Together they're essential to healthy nerve tissue and to the body's conversion of food into energy. When you exercise strenuously, your body uses up its vitamin B resources in short order and performance deteriorates. Unfortunately, B vitamins are particularly delicate—they're lost quickly when foods are cooked, processed, or even just stored. Even with foods that are said to be rich in B complex, it's impossible in today's American grocery or restaurant to know what you're really getting.

B_1 (thiamine) is crucial to the breakdown of carbohydrates and the release of energy. Food refining robs carbohydrates of this nutrient—white flour and white sugar are among the worst offenders. Whole grains, wheat germ, bran, and raw sunflower seeds are fairly dependable natural sources.

B_2 (riboflavin) appears to help release energy from fats. In addition, new or damaged tissues need riboflavin to build and repair themselves; B_2 can speed up muscle building and help heal torn ligaments. More Americans, about one in three, are deficient in B_2 than any other vitamin. Dairy products, leafy vegetables, and beef liver are good sources, but canning, cooking, and even exposing these foods to light can seriously diminish their riboflavin content.

B_3 (niacin) is especially important to the athlete because it helps to dilate blood vessels and promote oxygen transport through the body. This means that sufficient niacin keeps you from getting exhausted so quickly. In addition, vitamin B_3 serves as an enzyme in breaking down carbohydrates and comes into play in several stages of your body's energy cycle. Poultry, fish, lean meats, and peanuts when very fresh, contain high levels of B_3.

B_5 (pantothenic acid) is sometimes called the *antistress vitamin* because it helps keep your adrenal glands in working order, and they in turn regulate your body's metabolism and reaction to stress. Physical exertion is one form of stress that uses up large amounts of B_5. Studies have shown that pantothenic acid can increase endurance and tolerance to the cold. Organ meats, egg yolks, and sunflower seeds usually provide B_5 in abundance.

B_6 (pyridoxine) facilitates the conversion of stored liver and muscle glycogen into energy, as well as helping your body utilize amino acids and protein. The more protein you eat, the more pyridoxine you need. Look to liver, white chicken meat, fish, whole grains, bananas, and raw nuts and seeds for a steady supply of this vitamin. As always, these sources are reliable only when *fresh*, and these days the only way to be completely certain of freshness is to harvest your own vegetables and slaughter your own animals.

B_{12} (cobalamin) is important in the formation of DNA. Its deficiency causes a failure of cellular maturation and division, and also inhibits the rate of red blood cell production. For years athletes have taken liver tablets for their B_{12} content. This practice stemmed from the belief that B_{12} improves energy, although it seems unlikely unless a preexisting deficiency exists. It's referred to as the antipernicious anemia vitamin, a condition in which B_{12} is digested before it can be absorbed into the bloodstream. B_{12} is protected from this destructive digestion under normal circumstances by a gastric secretion called the intrinsic factor, which combines with the B_{12} until absorption occurs.

The richest sources for this vitamin are animal organ meats, but white fish, cheese, and eggs also contain high levels. Because your liver stores massive quantities of this vitamin (typically 300 times the RDA), your daily requirement for B_{12} is only about 3 micrograms. However, most commercially available supplements contain 100–300 micrograms.

Vitamin C

Hailed by some extremists as a miracle cure for everything from depression to the common cold, vitamin C (ascorbic acid) is a big mover and shaker. Without enough of it, you get tired rapidly, recover from injuries slowly, and fall victim to severe stress. Scurvy, a potentially fatal disease of bleeding gums and extreme weakness, represents the extreme case of vitamin C deprivation.

Ascorbic acid helps you get the most out of your muscles in a variety of ways. It aids muscle tissue in utilizing fatty acids as an energy source, thereby conserving glycogen, the major fuel, and adding to endurance. C helps your body use iron and oxygen efficiently while protecting other vitamins from harmful oxygenation. Recent research also indicates that vitamin C slows down lactic acid buildup during exertion, thereby minimizing fatigue. Also, like B_6, vitamin C protects your body against the harmful effects of stress by keeping the adrenal glands working.

Vitamin C's primary role is as biochemical partner in the formation and maintenance of collagen, the protein "cement" that binds connective tissue. Collagen holds together muscles, skin, bones, organs—literally your whole body. Athletes recovering from injuries, especially after surgery, use up vast amounts of this nutrient.

You should pay particular attention to maintaining your stores of vitamin C. Stress, as well as steroids, aspirin, and smoking, rapidly deplete your levels of ascorbic acid. Oranges are probably the best-known natural source of vitamin C—ships that set out to sea take cases of them along to prevent sailors from getting scurvy—but surprisingly this fruit can't be relied on; some oranges have plenty of ascorbic acid, while others have only trace levels. Even eating a dozen oranges a day can't guarantee you'll get your daily requirement. Supplements seem to be the only solution.

Vitamin D

Sunshine on yeast produces vitamin D (cholecalciferol), hence the name, "sunshine vitamin." The now well-known deficiency diseases associated with this vitamin are rickets (in children) and osteomalacia (in adults). In both diseases there is a softening of the bones because of a lack of calcium phosphate.

Sun shining on the face alone will produce 10 micrograms (in winter only about 1 microgram) after three hours of exposure. Total body exposure will produce up to 100 micrograms in that period of time.

Since the recommended daily allowance for vitamin D is only 5 micrograms, it's rare that vitamin D needs to be taken in supplement form. Because it can be toxic in doses exceeding 10 micrograms (equivalent to 40 International Units), supplementation should only be done in periods when you are not exposed to sunshine for more than about three hours per day, especially during the winter months.

Some of the toxicity symptoms are: loss of appetite, nausea, constant thirst, headaches, and loss of weight, irritability and depression (in children).

Vitamin E

Vitamin E is the name given to a number of related viscous oils that work to keep your cardiovascular system clear and dilated, thus increasing the blood supply to your extremities. This nutrient also protects muscle and nerve tissue from overoxygenation while at the same time enabling your muscles to get by on less oxygen; so it promotes endurance. Athletes working out in high elevations, where oxygen is thin, can benefit particularly from a vitamin E supplement. Some doctors even recommend E as a treatment for acne. Wheat germ, whole grains, raw seeds, nuts, and soybeans contain high levels of this vitamin.

Vitamin K

Vitamin K's sole function is to control the rate of blood clotting. A deficiency for this vitamin will cause several other symptoms to occur including liver disease, malabsorption of fats, low bile salt formation, and excessive bleeding if bruised or wounded.

Since healthy people manufacture adequate vitamin K in the intestines (through activity of intestinal bacteria), it is rarely necessary to supplement your diet with this vitamin. However, no toxicity symptoms have been recorded, and you can safely supplement with up to 1000 micrograms or more per day. The best sources for vitamin K are cauliflower, brussels sprouts, and broccoli, but lettuce, spinach, cabbage, and tomatoes have high levels also.

Minerals

For a long time, vitamins had the spotlight as necessities for good health, but the role of minerals, which may be even more crucial, emerged only with recent advances in biochemistry. If you're deficient in minerals, the consequences are dire: any body lacking even one mineral can't function properly. Minerals combine with vitamins to form enzymes involved in almost every physiological process.

Minerals can be found in a wide range of plant and animal foods, as well as in drinking water, but too often the quantities are insufficient. As an athlete, you need to be particularly careful to maintain adequate mineral levels because the stress of exercise rapidly depletes your body's stores. Serious deficiencies, especially of iron and calcium, are disturbingly common among otherwise healthy Americans, with women more susceptible than men. If you're prone to injury, fatigue, or sluggishness, you may well be one of these individuals.

Calcium

A silvery, metallic element in natural form, calcium is the most abundant mineral in the human body. Besides helping to make up bones and teeth, it's necessary for triggering muscle contraction in your heart, lungs, arms, and legs, especially.

Although calcium can be found in milk, cheese, salad greens, and many fortified processed foods, possibly half the women and nearly as many men in this country don't get enough of it. According to Dr. Cogan, your body absorbs only about one-tenth of the calcium in dairy products.

"That's why you see so many athletes with stress fractures," Colgan says. "The bones are put under enormous stress, without the raw materials being provided." The more often your body undergoes the stress of impact—for example, in running, jumping, and contact sports—the more crucial calcium becomes. Colgan advocates plentiful calcium supplements, calcium carbonate in particular.

Magnesium

Sweating drains more magnesium from your body than any other mineral. Whereas calcium facilitates muscular contraction, magnesium is intimately involved in the process of relaxation, as well as in the digestion of meat. Fatigue, spasms, twitching, and muscular weakness are all symptoms of a magnesium shortage. Processed foods are again responsible for the lack of magnesium in the American diet. It can, however, still be found in whole grains, such as whole wheat and brown rice, as well as in leafy vegetables, soybeans, corn, apples, seeds, and nuts.

Dr. Colgan says the RDA for magnesium is too low to sustain athletic activity. The commonly suggested ratio for calcium to magnesium is two to one, but Colgan thinks four to three is more like it, which means you should take 1,000 milligrams of calcium for every 750 milligrams of magnesium supplements.

Phosphorus

Phosphorus, second only to calcium in its abundance in your body, plays a crucial role in many biochemical reactions. The mineral enables you to utilize the food you eat, and as a component of adenosine triphosphate, it's involved in every muscular contraction. Great, right? Well, the problem in most diets is too much of a good thing.

Phosphorus causes depletion of calcium and magnesium in bones, muscles, and organs, so the symptom of overabundant phosphorus is the same as for insufficiency of the other two minerals, namely weakness. The recommended balance between phosphorus and calcium is one to one; meats and poultry contain a ratio of 20 to one. Even worse in this regard are carbonated soft drinks, commercial baked goods (including cake mixes), processed and cured meats, potato chips, and many salad dressings. Beyond avoiding these foods, your solution is supplements of calcium and magnesium.

Sodium and Potassium

You need a proper balance of these two minerals (1:1) to achieve maximum muscular power. Sodium and potassium are necessary for transmitting nerve impulses; if you're lacking in either or if the ratio is imbalanced, you'll suffer from cramping and weakness.

It's easy to overdose on sodium in this country. Typical American use of table salt can jack up your sodium level to more than 10 times the minimum requirement. This makes it unlikely that you'll deplete your supply by sweating. Salt tablets, which athletes used to consume by the handful, can do a great deal more harm than good by diverting fluid away from working muscles and into the stomach to dilute the sodium. If you're sweating hard, drink water. Only if you're on a low-salt diet are you apt to suffer from sodium shortage during a hot-weather workout.

Because of oversalting in their diets, athletes are more likely to be in danger of being deficient in potassium. Besides supplements, leafy green vegetables, bananas, citrus, and dried fruits are good natural sources of potassium.

Iron

Without iron, your bloodstream would be incapable of carrying or storing oxygen; it's a critical part of both hemoglobin and myoglobin. A lack of iron is the most common of mineral deficiencies, afflicting nine out of 10 women and a great many men, irrespective of age, race, or income. Long-distance runners and other endurance athletes are particularly prone to iron shortages, which can result in the failure to make gains despite hard training.

Female athletes particularly need to monitor their iron levels and take supplements. Dried, unsulfured apricots and raisins, liver, and oysters are iron-rich; you can even bolster your levels by cooking in an iron pot. Coffee and tea can block the absorption of iron from food by as much as 80 percent, so avoid them if you think you might be one of the deficient many.

Zinc

Long neglected by nutritionists, zinc has recently come into its own as a mineral acknowledged to be critical to health. It helps A and B complex vitamins do their jobs, strengthens your immune system, and increases your stamina by prolonging muscle contraction. Keep zinc oxide ointment around for abrasions and wounds—applying it directly to the trouble site can help speed up the healing process.

Due to the overuse of chemical fertilizers and to grain-refining methods, much of the world's population has become zinc-deficient.

40

Oysters and eggs are strong sources, but a supplement is probably necessary in your diet.

Iodine

Before iodized salt was invented, there was a "goiter belt" in the central United States due to a lack of the dietary iodine that those on either coast got from seafood. Only one ten-thousandth of a gram of iodine per day is necessary for health, but low iodine levels (hypothyroidism) still persist because of inadequate absorption. Athletes need to take in iodine to ensure stamina. Seafood and iodized salt are excellent sources; if you're on a low-salt diet, be sure to make up for it with an iodine supplement.

Manganese

No one knows yet exactly how this mineral works, but no one doubts its benefits. Manganese must be present for coordinated muscular activity, and the mineral helps to heal injuries of bones, cartilage, tendons, and ligaments. Unrefined grains, oatmeal, and bananas provide the highest levels.

Daily Vitamin and Mineral Supplementation

The only way to be sure you're getting the nutrients you need is to take the appropriate supplements every day. As an athlete, you can bet you need a good deal more than the RDA. The vitamin market can be intimidating to the novice, however, offering a vast array of alternatives, not all of which are particularly healthful. Individual supplements contain anywhere from mini- to megadoses, while the multiples and packets each claim to give you all you need (hard to do, since everyone's needs differ).

It's well worth it, though, to learn the mysteries of vitamins and minerals and invest in the best you can buy. Give your body what it needs, and it will pay you back 10-fold with superior performance.

The following table lists all the essential vitamin and mineral RDAs for men and women, and the ranges of dosages typically found in commercially available supplements.

Perhaps the most convenient way to take vitamin and mineral supplements is the daily pack. Almost all major vitamin manufacturers nowadays provide all of the vitamins and minerals you need daily in one small cellophane package for easy use. You won't have to open dozens of bottles each morning to get your daily quotas. Most such multivitamin/mineral packs come in a box supplying you with one month's supply.

Be sure to read the label, however, and avoid those which provide

Supplementing with Vitamins and Trace Elements			
Substance	US RDA (1980) Male 23–50	US RDA (1980) Female 23–50	Ranges Used For Supplements (per day)
Retinol/Beta-carotene	1,000 mcg RE	800 mcg RE	1,000–9,000 mcg RE
Thiamine	1.4 mg	1.0 mg	40–600 mg
Riboflavin	1.6 mg	1.2 mg	30–250 mg
Niacin/Niacinamide	18 mg	13 mg	100–1,000 mg
Pantothenic acid			50–1,000 mg
Pyridoxine	2.2 mg	2.0 mg	40–300 mg
Cobalamins	3.0 mcg	3.0 mcg	100–300 mcg
Folacin	400 mcg	400 mcg	2–30 mg
Biotin			2–100 mg
Inositol			100–1,000 mg
P-Amino-benzoic acid			100–500 mg
Phosphatidyl choline			200–2,000 mg
Ascorbates	60 mg	60 mg	2,000–16,000 mg
Cholecalciferol	5 mcg	5 mcg	5–62 mcg
Tocopherols	10 mg TE	8 mg TE	200–1,600 mg TE
Zinc	15 mg	15 mg	50–150 mg
Iron	10 mg	18 mg	30–60 mg
Iodine	150 mcg	150 mcg	0.15–1.0 mg
Calcium	800 mg	800 mg	1,000–3,500 mg
Magnesium	350 mg	300 mg	1,000–2,000 mg
Manganese			20–100 mg
Phosphorus	800 mg	800 mg	200–2,000 mg
Potassium			198–5,000 mg
Copper			0–5 mg
Molybdenum			50–500 mcg
Chromium			0.3–1.0 mg
Selenium			0.2–1.0 mg

Here are the National Research Council's Recommended Dietary Allowances for men and women as they compare to a more useful range of daily intakes, which appears in the far right column. If you're active and train vigorously, the amount of vitamins and minerals you probably need is more likely to fall within that range. Some essential elements aren't used here, or are used in very tiny quantities, bcause most people have ample amounts in their diets or tissues. (Beta carotene is usually converted into retinol equivalents—REs—and tocopherols of vitamin E to tocopherol equivalents, or TEs.)

potentially toxic levels of the fat-soluble vitamins (A, D, E). Also avoid manufacturers who make unsubstantiated claims regarding their product's superiority because of its higher doses. Instead, stick to those products that provide at *least* the RDAs of each substance *plus* a reasonable margin beyond for athletes' increased needs.

The real value of vitamin/mineral supplements lies not in their ability to produce instant performance or energy improvements. They simply cannot do that unless there has been a deficiency beforehand (often likely). Instead, their real value is in taking them religiousiy—on a daily basis—over the course of several months.

Chapter 9 ("The Role of Supplements") explains the significance of careful vitamin/mineral supplementation. Given the state of the art in nutritional biochemistry, it's difficult (if not impossible) to pinpoint exact vitamin and mineral needs of athletes. Instead, we resort appropriately to a controlled "shotgun" approach, ensuring that our daily needs are exceeded by a safe margin. This is a safe approach, and one which works well over the course of months of training.

8
FOOD ALLERGIES AND FOOD INTOLERANCES

Say you eat some wheat, and soon your nose is running, your eyes are puffed, and you're overcome with sleepiness. What's more, the same symptoms seem to occur every time you eat that food. What you could be experiencing is a health disorder known as a *food allergy.*

We're hearing a lot more about food allergies these days, and the condition must be taken seriously by athletes, because adverse reactions to certain foods can wreak havoc with your training (see list at the end of this chapter). If you find that certain foods cause discomfort such as nausea and headaches, you obviously are going to have to plan your Ultimate Sports Nutrition program around them.

Doing so can be a challenge sometimes because, as luck would have it, some of the main suspected allergens are among the most popular foods for athletes: wheat, seafood, nuts, tomatoes, berries, and citrus fruits, as well as milk, eggs, chocolate, and spices. Having a bad reaction to these or other foods does *not* mean that there's necessarily anything wrong with the foods. It doesn't even mean that you should cut them out. Many adverse reactions that people are quick to call "allergies" really aren't.

A true food allergy is an immunological reaction, meaning that certain components of your body's immune system must be activated. The main defense against invasion by viruses or bacteria, the immune system sometimes overreacts to certain substances in certain individuals—that reaction is what we call an *allergy*.

Food allergies usually occur within 30 to 45 minutes after eating. The symptoms include itching or swelling in the mouth, hives, skin swelling, nausea, vomiting, headache, sinusitis, diarrhea, cystitis, general fatigue, and behavioral abnormalities.

46

Food Additives

Asthmatics notice more than most people that certain food additives can cause allergic reactions. Within 30 minutes of ingesting certain additives, they experience full-blown asthma attacks.

The main offender is a coloring agent called *tartarizine* (also known as "F, D and C Yellow 5"). A number of people are also sensitive to sulfites—sulfur dioxide and potassium- or sodium-metabisulfite—which are used to preserve foods such as shrimp, peeled and processed potatoes, and salad bar vegetables. Beer, wine, and champagne also contain sulfites.

Both tartarizine and sulfites are on the Food and Drug Administration's GRAS ("Generally Recognized as Safe") list, but that clearly doesn't mean that those additives can't cause adverse reactions in some people. They do.

Remember, then, if you notice allergic manifestations when eating certain foods, check for additives before condemning the food itself. Keep in mind that what's "GRAS" for some may not be for you.

Dealing With Food Allergies

Doctors use a number of tests to find suspected food allergens, including skin tests and radioallergosorbent testing (RAST), which detects the presence of an antibody (Immunoglobin E) that's always found in larger amounts in allergic individuals. In recent years, there's been a lot of media hype for so-called "cytotoxic testing," which involves isolating white blood cells and testing their reaction to suspected food allergens.

Cytotoxic testing appeals to many people, athletes included, because of cure-all promises. The problem is that there's no valid proof that it works. The tests often fail to uncover foods to which an individual may be allergic, and they're plagued by false positive and false negative results.

Probaby the most reliable method of ascertaining food allergies is the elimination diet. It's tedious, but it works. If you experience allergic reactions, eliminate all suspected food allergens from your diet. Then, keeping a meticulous food diary in which you note every crumb that enters your mouth, add the foods back one by one. The culprit will be apparent when the allergic symptoms return.

If you're one of the unfortunate athletes who reacts allergically to certain foods, remember that no food is indispensable. If you need to eliminate a key food from your diet because of food allergies, replace the nutrient with another food source or by taking supplements.

47

For example, if you have a problem with milk, such as lactose intolerance, cut out milk from your diet and replace the missing calcium and protein with supplements of other foods containing those nutrients, such as leafy green vegetables, soy nuts, citrus fruits, sardines and salmon with their bones, oysters, and tofu.

Food allergies are bad for your training and complicate your nutrition program. But you don't have to be the victim of hucksters peddling cytotoxic testing to set things right.

Food Intolerance

Not to be confused with allergies, food intolerance is a much broader term. Intolerances to certain foods can manifest themselves in several ways and do not register on traditional allergy tests.

Typical reasons why some people develop intolerances to certain foods are enzyme deficiencies (resulting in the inability to fully digest certain foods) and antibiotics use (which can kill certain "good" bacteria in the intestinal tract). Some chemicals (caffeine and food additives such as tartarazine) can also cause an intolerance to the foods containing them.

In practice, however, allergies and intolerances are often treated the same—through the elimination diet plan. It makes little difference whether an immune response or an intolerance is responsible for your discomfort. The result is the same—poor training.

Symptoms to look for include the following if you suspect an allergy or an intolerance.

spastic colon (diarrhea, abdominal pain, abdominal distension)
migraine headache (usually on one side of the head, often accompanied by nausea or vomiting)
rhinitis (runny nose, stuffiness, often chronic, lasting for weeks)

asthma (wheezing, shortness of breath, nocturnal coughing)

gluten sensitive enteropathy (damaged intestinal lining from gluten, a protein found in wheat; can lead to diarrhea, bone disease, stunted growth, weight loss or anemia)

eczema (scaly or crusty skin, often on elbows or knees)

urticaria (large red blotches, often causing itching, swollen lips)

arthritis (inflammation of the joints stemming from osteoarthritis [wear and tear, not affected by diet]; gout [caused by uric acid crystals forming in the joints as a result of purine-rich foods such as organ meats, peas, beans, sardines and anchovies]; and rheumatoid arthritis [joints of the extremities, may or may not be linked to diet])

hyperactivity (overactivity symptomatology includes poor eating habits, abnormal thirst, learning disabilities, headaches, pollen allergies and nasal discharge; normally occurs in boys aged one to seven; often traced to foods and substances such as additives, aspirin, antural salicylates in some fruits and vegetables, dust, chemical aerosols, disinfectants, and perfumes)

It's clear that many of the foods and products commonly found in every home can be the root of allergies or sensitivities. If you suspect such to be the case, and if it's interfering with your health, fitness, or sports performance goals, the best advice I can give you is to see a medical doctor specializing in such problems, and the chances are that an exclusion diet will be recommended.

PART THREE
SUPPLEMENTS TO GOOD NUTRITION

9
THE ROLE OF SUPPLEMENTS

Now that you have a basic understanding of your needs concerning protein, carbohydrates, fats, vitamins, and minerals, it's time to ask the important question: How do supplements fit into your Ultimate Sports Nutrition program?

Nutritional supplementation for athletes in training is a science. But as I pointed out earlier, the debate has been dominated by extremists and curmudgeons with little understanding of the requirements of athletes. Only recently have some intrepid sleuths of academe begun offering some relevant research results.

And God bless those folks! It does my heart good to thumb my nose at proponents of all foolish and potentially danerous extremes. The no-dose and megadose fruitcakes can go fight their battles in outer space, where they belong.

Here's the truth about what constitutes sound nutrition for athletes: *Nutritional supplements usually, but not always, are necessary.*

You don't need protein supplements when you're not training hard. And you don't need vitamin and mineral supplements when you're eating three or four perfectly balanced meals per day.

You probably don't fit into either one of those categories. No athlete I know has ever achieved any success without training regularly. And I've never met a soul anywhere who eats properly all the time. Even if you tried, obtaining all of your nutritional requirements in the form of food is nothing but a pipe dream in today's compromised environment.

So I conclude that supplementing your diet is necessary most of the time for athletes. As in anything else concerning your diet, knowledge is power. To determine how much to supplement and what to supplement with, you must apply the information in the following chapters to the reason you eat as an athlete and to the basic nutritional requirements discussed in Part II.

Nutritional supplements are not drugs. They can't produce a quick psychological or physiological fix. All nutrients act slowly, as generations of old cells die and are replaced by new and improved cells in the enriched nutrient medium.

That gradual process is one of the reasons that scientific studies haven't been much help in designing an optimum nutritional supplementation program that will aid athletes in achieving peak performance. They've been of short duration, even though to be valid and useful nutritional studies should be at least 20 weeks long. It takes 18 to 20 weeks, for example, for new blood cells to completely replace old ones. And it takes years for a proper nutritional program to build an optimal body.

There are two other big reasons why a general effective supplementation program for athletes is so illusive. One is that most studies have used only one nutrient at a time—or an arbitrary combination of a few nutrients—rather than a comprehensive nutritional approach that permits synergistic interreactions of the ingredients. The other is that previous studies have failed to take into account the biochemical differences in individuals and the resultant differences in their nutritional requirements.

Remember the table in Chapter 2 that listed the many variables that determine an individual athlete's nutritional needs? One of those variables is *physiological dynamics*, which refers to the fact that it takes a varying amount of time—but at least several months—for a nutritional supplementation program to produce physiological changes. Of course, that's why short-lived studies of the effects of supplements are fruitless. It's also something for you to remember as you gauge the effects of supplementation on your nutrition program.

An illuminating study in this regard was performed by Dr. Colgan, the sports nutritionist. Marathon runners fed vitamin and

51

Comparison Data for the Two Marathon Groups

	Subject	Age	No. of previous marathons or races of 20+ miles	Best marathon time (hrs:min:sec)	Marathon time at conclusion of study (hrs:min:sec)	Improvement (min:sec)
Experimental Group (Vitamin and mineral supplements)	E1	28	7	2:31:40	2:21:56	9:44
	E2	30	18	2:53:20	2:38:02	17:18
	E3	38	6	2:59:17	2:30:52	28:25
	E4	44	25	2:48:01	2:33:31	15:30
					Mean improvement	17:44
Control Group (No supplements)	C1	29	6	2:36:18	2:27:48	8:30
	C2	32	9	2:52:00	2:57:03	(-5:03)
	C3	35	11	2:55:23	2:48:22	7:01
	C4	42	19	2:50:35	2:39:15	11:20
					Mean improvement (taking C2 as zero)	6:43

Source: Colgan, M. Effects of multi-nutrient supplementation on athletic performance. *Proceedings of the 1984 Olympic Scientific Congress* (ed. Katch, F. I.), Human Kinetics Publishers, Champaign, IL, 1984.

mineral supplements experienced nearly three times as much performance improvement as their control group counterparts after about six months of training, as the preceding table shows. I regard this study and others like it as compelling evidence that supplementation is not only beneficial but *necessary* for peak athletic performance.

10
AMINO ACIDS AS SUPPLEMENTS

You already know the critical role that protein plays in an athlete's muscle development and health. And you know that amino acids are the building blocks of protein.

But they're much more than that. Research has shown that proper amino acid supplementation can be as effective as anabolic steroids in building muscle and strength—*without* the health risks, legal problems, and moral questions associated with steroids.

What Are Amino Acids?

Technically, amino acids are organic compounds that have both an amino (NH_2) and a carboxyl (COOH) radical in their structure. The amino acids found in protein are categorized in two groups: *essential* amino acids and *nonessential* amino acids—a misleading term because all of the amino acids are essential. Those that aren't manufactured by the body (or are manufactured only in very small amounts) are the so-called essential amino acids and so have to be derived from food.

The *essential* amino acids are threonine, lysine, methionine, arginine (for children and athletes), valine, phenylalanine, leucine, tryptophan, isoleucine, and histidine (for children and athletes). The *nonessential* amino acids are glycine, alanine, serine, cysteine, aspartic acid, glutamic acid, norleucine, beta-hydroxyglutamic acid, cystine, tyrosine, proline, and hydroxyproline.

To complicate the picture, there are certain amino acids not present in protein that have found their way into the pharmaceutical gym bag of many athletes. One in particular is *L.3—dihydroxyphenylalanine* or *L-Dopa*. L-Dopa is a potent stimulator of human growth hormone (HGH), but it has some serious side effects and should be avoided.

Another HGH-stimulating amino acid not found in protein is *5-hydroxytryptophan*. It too has side effects, so arginine and ornithine (another amino acid not found in muscle) are frequently substituted because they are apparently safe as well as reasonably effective HGH stimulators. So too are *lysine, cysteine, tryptophan,* and *histidine*, a derivative of arginine. The growth hormone stimulation effect has opened up a whole new field of nutritional supplementation.

Protein cannot be manufactured by the body unless all of the required amino acids are present. In fact, all of the amino acids must be at the site of protein synthesis before any of them can act. If some are not present when needed, those that are present either get stored or are degraded by the liver and used as energy or stored as fat.

Clearly, amino acids exert a profound effect on our overall health and physical performance. Indeed, the amino acid cycles (processes) basically run the body. For these cycles to work properly, it's important that the amino acids be in the right proportion. Also, many of the cycles are vitamin- and mineral-dependent, which means the process will be impaired if a particular vitamin or mineral isn't present in sufficient quantity. For example, the amino acid methionine is dependent on vitamin B_6 and magnesium; the methionine cycle won't work unless there is sufficient vitamin B_6 and magnesium in the body.

Amino acid supplementation is mandatory for any athlete who wishes to maximize performance (and teenage athletes, incidentally, have greater amino acid requirements than adults). But *you can't take amino acids haphazardly*. The body is a delicate balance of interacting chemical reactions. Since amino acids are intimately involved in many of these, imbalances can occur if additions are made at key points in the reaction sequence. Such imbalances not only can make an amino acid supplementation program useless for energy production, for example, but can actually result in a *loss* of energy—hardly what a serious athlete wants!

There are only a few laboratories in the country that perform a new analytical technique measuring levels of amino acids in the body. This is done primarily by means of a urine test. The urine specimen can be mailed to the lab, so the athlete does not have to leave home to have the analysis performed. On some occasions the doctors will resort to a blood analysis as a backup measure if the urine test results are inconclusive. The urine test is preferred, however, since urine is the end product of metabolism.

Following the test, the athlete is put on an appropriate amino acid supplementation regimen and periodically retested to determine if there are imbalances in the individual's amino acid cycles. Here are two labs to contact for amino acid analysis (always consult your sports medicine physician on matters of urine or blood analysis procedures and interpretation of the results): MetaMetrix Laboratories, Inc., Atlanta, GA (urinalysis kit provided via mail with instructions for return mailing of sample) and Tyson Laboratories, Inc., Santa Monica, CA (blood test results from your personal physician are required for analysis). Both companies make recommendations from their analysis regarding your need for certain amino acids, and offer to provide you with them—they both manufacture and sell amino acid supplements.

Obviously, this procedure yields an enormous amount of information on the athlete's metabolic processes, which allows the scientists to pinpoint problem areas and fine-tune the diet and supplement regimen to optimize physical performance.

To see how amino acid analysis works, let's look at a couple of case studies.

Case Studies

Case Study 1

A 40-year-old karate instructor, highly conditioned from working out several hours a day, complained of chronic sinus drainage and loss of muscle mass. He could not gain weight no matter how much he ate—and he said a typical dinner might include 12 pieces of chicken or a large steak!

An amino acid analysis revealed a primary digestive problem. Subsequent testing showed low stomach acidity, but high acidity in the small intestine. This combination can dramatically reduce one's ability to digest protein. The incomplete protein digestion led to the formation of a metabolic by-product that caused his kidneys to excrete excessive amounts of amino acids in the urine. This caused an eventual loss of muscle mass as his body literally began to feed on itself for the protein to supply the vital organs. The incomplete protein digestion also was causing chronic food allergies, which he experienced as sinus problems.

Here was a man, who, ironically, was losing body protein (muscle) because he was consuming too much food protein (meat). Solution? A low-protein, high-carbohydrate diet with supplementation of free-form amino acids, digestive aids, and certain vitamins and minerals that the analysis indicated he required for optimal amino acid metabolism. Since meats were eliminated from the diet, the man's body no longer made the by-product that caused the protein loss. The free-form amino acids, which did not require digestion, were readily absorbed and utilized by the body.

In two weeks the man gained five pounds, which he felt was muscle mass, and the sinus problems disappeared. He also reported that he was in a much better mood and no longer felt burnt out at the end of the day.

Case Study 2

A 20-year-old competitive bodybuilder had been regularly using anabolic steroids and following the high-protein, low-carbohydrate diet so popular among strength athletes. He wasn't experiencing any problems; he simply was looking for a training boost prior to an important competition.

After a complete amino acid analysis, it was determined that he needed a dramatic change in his diet and a supplementation regimen. He promptly went on a low-protein, high-carbohydrate diet tailored to his metabolism and started taking a special amino acid formulation between meals and before workouts. The supplements were designed specifically to stimulate energy metabolism and enhance protein in the muscles during a workout.

His progress was so good that he discontinued using steroids. While the muscle mass of his competitors decreased as they dieted severely to get lean and defined in the last few weeks before the contest, this young athlete's muscles continued to grow! He gained 10 pounds of lean body mass in the three weeks before the competition, and his body fat percentage dropped from 10 percent to 8 percent. He experienced increased energy and less lactic acid burn at high reps in his training sessions. His muscles pumped up better—and the pumps lasted longer.

This bodybuilder now is determined to reach the top without

using steroids. Cases like this hold promise that the present dependence on steroids in sports can be eliminated. It's my view that, through proper biochemical analysis, diet, and supplementation, the body can be maximally stimulated to optimal performance without drugs and their negative side effects.

Taking Amino Acids

- *It's extremely important to supplement the diet with vitamin B_6.* Today, fruits and vegetables have excessive pesticide residue that cannot be washed off. Ingesting these pesticides (which is unavoidable), apparently creates an increased physiological need for vitamin B_6. Since a B_6 deficiency in the body will seriously interfere with amino acid cycles, it's recommended that the diet be supplemented with 100–300 milligrams of vitamin B_6 each day.

- *Athletes should not take the amino acids arginine and ornithine in high doses (2,000 or more milligrams per day).* Despite what Durk Pearson and Sandy Shaw say in their best-selling book *Life Extension*, supplementing with these amino acids is not the last word. Large doses of arginine and ornithine throw off the amino acid metabolism. It's also known that taking large amount of arginine causes an increased susceptibility to oral herpes. For best result, take these amino acids in small quantities (1200 milligrams/day).

- *When supplementing the diet with vitamins, pass on the vitamin D.* Tests show that vitamin D can affect amino acid cycles in the body. If you're taking a multivitamin, choose one that has a low amount of D—no higher than the RDA.

- *People on high-protein diets tend to be protein-starved. Paradoxically, those on a high-carbohydrate diet generally have a much better amino acid balance.* Over the years, it's been customary for athletes to think, "If I want to excel in my sport, if I want to become big and strong, I must eat more protein—specifically, animal protein." Yes, there seems to be a certain logic in football players, wrestlers, bodybuilders, weightlifters, and boxers making meat the main course of their diet. After all, these strength athletes are the "lions" of the sports world, and who ever heard of lions sitting down to a meal of nuts, fruits, and vegetables?

Yet, when biochemical analysis is done, revealing how well the body is functioning, that traditional, seemingly logical theory of sports nutrition just doesn't hold up. The direct feedback from athletes on a high-protein diet (consisting of more than two grams of protein per kilogram of body weight per day) is that they are very unhealthy, tend to suffer from nutritional allergies, have problems with their kidneys and other organs, and—remarkably—are protein-starved (as was the case with the karate instructor mentioned earlier).

Scientists in Georgia tested athletes who were taking in more than 2 grams per kilogram of body weight of animal protein a day, but whose bodies were assimilating only about 30 grams. These individuals actually were losing muscle weight and strength because they were intolerant to that excessive amount of protein. Their bodies were not able to break it down. If you take in too much protein, the body gets to a point where it actually seems to turn off the assimilating process, as if to say, "Hey, you're putting in too much; I can't handle it. There's too much for me to break down and detoxify. So, forget it, I'm shutting down."

As far as amino acid analysis is concerned, no one seriously would suggest that such testing is imperative for everyone active in sports. The weekend or recreational athlete really doesn't need to worry about body chemistry and maximum performance. Most serious athletes may not see a need for sophisticated biochemical testing either. For such individuals, a basically sound diet (minimum 70 percent carbohydrate, with 1.2–1.8 grams of protein per kilogram of body weight per day), daily vitamin-mineral supplementation, and a careful, intelligent amino acid program (high in branch-chain amino acids, i.e., a formula specially designed for athletes) should serve the nutritional needs adequately.

But at the elite level in athletics, sophisticated bioanalytic techniques such as amino acid analysis are important, if not imperative. After all, athletic performance has entered the high-tech age. And it hardly makes sense to use highly scientific training techniques and the most advanced equipment while leaving one's nutrition up to chance.

So the elite modern athlete intent on maximizing performance can—and should—take steps to ensure that the body is biochemically correct and balanced. It's important to check whether the thyroid, adrenal glands, and liver are functioning properly. Is there a sufficient amount of vitamins and minerals in the body? Most important of all, it's crucial for such an athlete to make sure there are no blocks in any of the amino acid cycles, the metabolic pathways in the body.

How do you make sure there are no blocks? The only way to find out is by undergoing an amino acid analysis.

What Do Amino Acids Do?

Branched-Chain Amino Acids

Thirty-five percent of your muscles are made up of the amino acids leucine, isoleucine, and valine. They are known as *branched-chain amino acids* because of their molecular configuration. These three amino acids must be present for muscular growth and development to take place. A deficiency in any one of them will result in muscle loss.

If your level of isoleucine is low (as detected in the urine), you'll typically have symptoms similar to hypoglycemia, such as listlessness, because the amino acid is important in converting muscle glycogen into energy. Since isoleucine is a major muscle builder, any deficiency can cause muscle mass losses.

Leucine is also important in muscle building, preventing muscle breakdown, and promoting healing. Low urine levels of leucine may indicate either a deficiency in your diet or a vitamin B_6 deficiency. Vitamin B_6 is a necessary factor in the enzyme system that is responsible for energy production and protein synthesis, and it's fundamental to the proper metabolism of valine. Low urine levels of valine can reflect either a B_6 deficiency or a low dietary intake of balanced protein (that is, the presence of all the essential amino acids). It is wise to supplement with additional valine even if your dietary protein intake is normal.

Histidine

Histidine is vital to the metabolic process of protein synthesis. The level of this amino acid in your urine reflects the general status of your muscle system. Low levels of histidine also have been linked to rheumatoid arthritis.

Arginine

Arginine is widely used by athletes as an agent in stimulating growth hormone release—the benefits of which are clearly controversial at this time. No one has conclusively shown that the small increase in the level of systemic growth hormone has a measurable anabolic, or tissue-building, effect. In fat, the use of arginine as an anabolic agent is so widespread that high levels—which often indicate ammonia toxicity in the body—are being observed in the urine of heavy users. Ammonia is formed by excessive urea production—too much protein or too many amino acids in the diet. A low-protein diet is recommended along with increased water intake.

Still, many proponents claim that measurable benefits to muscle development can be derived from arginine supplementation, but prudence and monitoring are essential.

Glycine

Glycine is the smallest amino acid. It serves as the basic nitrogen pool for the manufacture of the nonessential amino acids and is an important element in the structure of red blood cells. It's often used clinically in controlling depression. Creatine, an important source of muscular energy, requires glycine in the synthesis process, as do glucose and RNA and DNA. The most noticeable glycine deficiency symptom is a loss of energy.

Lysine

Low lysine levels can cause a slowdown in protein synthesis, affecting both muscle and collagen formation. Lysine and vitamin C together form L-carnitine, which enables your muscle cells to use oxygen. That makes lysine an invaluable supplement for endurance athletes.

Proline

Proline, like lysine, is used in the formation of collagen. High levels of this amino acid in your urine often indicate connective tissue damage. Proline can also be metabolized for muscular energy, and if you've got a deficiency you may suffer from fatigue.

Cystine

Cystine is thought to be a major component of tissue antioxidant mechanics, although the idea of antioxidants and their function in the body is still in its theoretical stages. As the theory goes, free radicals—tiny, toxic chemical fragments—are breathed, ingested, or formed within our bodies. These substances are credited with the ability to damage tissues and cells via some form of electrocution process, causing premature aging, lowered stamina, lowered energy, and reduced healing, among other things. Some speculate that substances or atoms called *radicals* somehow combine with oxygen and are transformed into free radicals. Thus, an antioxidant is a substance (notably vitamins E and C, some food additives and preservatives, and certain drugs) that prevents radicals from being transformed into a free-radical state. The theoretical benefits of cystine supplementation are improved healing, diminished pain from inflammation, prolonged youthfulness, less inflammation following injury, and stronger connective tissue.

Glutamic Acid

Glutamic acid is an important metabolic factor in energy production. It works in concert with several other nutritional components, including vitamin B_6, niacin (B_3), and magnesium.

Alanine

Alanine is an energy producer, and it helps regulate your blood sugar levels. It's synthesized in your muscle tissue from branched-chain amino acids and may be released into your urine during exercise. Chronic deficiencies of this amino acid may lead to muscle loss and poor glucose tolerance, but that may be avoided through supplementation with the branched-chain amino acids.

Serine

Serine, which is converted to cystine in your body, is an important element in producing cellular energy. Acetylcholine, an important meurotransmitter that aids memory and other parasympathetic functions of your body, requires serine as one of its critical components. Serine can be formed by the essential amino acid threonine. If you're deficient in serine, any supplement must also include vitamin B_6, magnesium, and phosphorus.

Threonine

As with arginine, excessive use of threonine can cause the formation of too much urea and consequently ammonia toxicity in your body. To be used effectively, threonine requires vitamin B_6, magnesium, and niacin. Both serine and glycine can be synthesized from this amino acid. A low energy level is often related to deficiencies of threonine.

62

Methionine

Methionine helps to remove poisonous wastes from your liver, assists in the regeneration of liver and kidney tissue, influences hair follicle health, and can be an effective antistress factor.

Phenylalanine

Phenylalanine is most active in the d,l,phenylalanine form, and is implicated in pain reduction and antidepression therapy. An entire chapter is devoted to this substance (Chapter 13).

Tryptophan

Tryptophan is known to cause secretion of a neurotransmitter substance in the brain called serotonin. Because of this it is a very effective sleep agent. Serotonin also helps to depress the ill effects of stress and moodiness, and is directly involved in regulating daily biological rhythms.

Aspartic Acid

Aspartic acid is involved in the conversion of carbohydrates into glucose and then into glycogen (called glycolysis), which is the chief source of muscle energy.

A User's Guide to Amino Acid Supplements

The complexity of your body's amino acid picture is matched only by the vast promise that additional research offers and the potential for improved fitness and athletic performance capabilities if amino acids are used accordingly. A careful analysis of your urine, and your blood in some cases, is the best way to determine whether you're deficient in or have an overabundance of any of the amino acids.

Haphazardly supplementing with these compounds could lead to impaired performance or toxicities. But with the guidance of a careful expert, your overall amino acid profile can provide you with a powerful tool in enhancing your energy level and muscle development.

As an athlete, you owe it to yourself to ask an important question: How can I improve my body's ability to build itself? In the past, building muscle mass, strength, stamina, and recuperative ability was often the domain of anabolic steroids, but that quick and easy way proved to have a lot of dangerous pitfalls. Today, every serious athlete knows that the answer lies in making these improvements naturally, and amino acids hold the key.

Many food supplement companies have jumped on the amino acid bandwagon in light of evidence suggesting that amino acids can deliver the performance boosts we all seek. But you *must* remember one crucial point. While amino acids can safely provide the size, strength, and endurance increases you want, their use and dosage should be determined carefully, with the guidance of a qualified specialist. If you make hasty, uninformed decisions about amino acid combination and frequency of doses, you can waste your money and produce little or no effect.

Ideally, you should have an amino acid analysis before you start supplementing, because testing is a whole new field, though it's difficult to obtain. (See information under "What Are Amino Acids?" in this chapter for labs specializing in amino acid analysis.) You can consult with a competent physiologist or nutritionist who's well versed in amino acid supplementation. Not all amino acid formulas work for everyone. The amount and combinations that are appropriate for you during one period of time may not be what you need at a later time because as your body's biochemistry changes so do your amino acid requirements. So those consultations should take place yearly or anytime you make a major change in training.

The Practical Use of Amino Acids

A good base formula should contain the following amino acids and nutrients: leucine, alanine, glutamic acid, glycine, lysine, proline, histidine, alpha ketoglutaric acid, L-carnitine, isoleucine, valine, cysteine, dimethyl glycine, arginine, bioun serine, pyridoxine, magnesium, and threonine. Some amino acids interfere with the effects of others, so it's important that your base formula doesn't include combinations of amino acids that inhibit one another. That's one of the reasons you need the advice of someone who's knowledgeable about amino acids. The exact quantities of each ingredient, as well as the ingredients themselves, vary widely in the commercially available brands of amino acid mixtures.

64

In conjunction with that base formula, you might want to consider some additional supplements:

- Serine may be taken between meals to increase blood sugar levels or before a workout or competition to generate energy. It's especially helpful if you have hypoglycemia.
- Alanine can also be taken between meals to increase the glycogen levels in your body, which protects your muscles. If you're under stress or have hypoglycemia, your body will break down muscle tissue to obtain the amino acids like alanine that it needs to raise the blood sugar level. I personally use it before workouts, between meals, and before bedtime. Dosages can be increased when you're under additional stress.
- Glutamic acid in powdered L-glutamine form helps memory and concentration. Personal experience with glutamine and medical exams in college showed that one to three grams of glutamine taken under the tongue every two hours was a good study aid. Glutamine is helpful if you're training intensely or involved in sports that require a great deal of concentration.
- Alpha ketoglutaric acid helps to drive your energy system and provides additional energy before training or competition.
- Carnitine helps to accelerate the fat-burning process by combining with fat and carrying it into the cells' mitochondria, where it's used for energy. This can result in lower body fat levels, increased long-term energy, and the ability to conduct more intense workouts.
- Citric aspartic acid, like alpha ketoglutaric acid, increases your available energy. It's especially helpful when taken before a workout or competition.
- Dimethyl glycine is excellent for boosting your immune system and for preventing or delaying the buildup of lactic acid in your muscles. It can prevent the painful muscle burn that occurs when you "hit the wall" or lift your maximum weight. In my opinion, it can give you the extra edge required of champions.

How to Take Amino Acids

As with all supplementation, you should start amino acid supplementation with small dosages and increase them gradually. You must also be taking a complete multivitamin and mineral supplement. Amino acids are dependent on vitamins and minerals to work.

Other important points to remember:

65

- The base amino acid formula should be taken after meals. You can take it between meals if you want to suppress your appetite, such as when you're dieting or (for bodybuilders) cutting up for competition. And you can also take it as a preworkout aid one-half hour before you take any other preworkout formula.
- Your body's biochemistry changes slowly. It may be 3 to 12 weeks before you see the full benefits of your supplementation program, although the initial response occurs within 36 to 48 hours.
- Overtraining, according to research, has a detrimental effect on amino acid metabolism, and I've also found that the majority of athletes I have observed have been guilty of overtraining. When the intensity of frequency of training is slowed down, there is a notable increase in muscle size, strength, and endurance. *Don't overtrain.* The key is *balance* between training and recovery time.
- Diet is very important. Animal proteins can limit amino acid response and therapy. The best diet consists of 60 to 70 percent complex carbohydrates, 10 to 20 percent animal protein, and 10 to 15 percent fats.

There are good reasons for these proportions. Carbohydrates spare the protein in your body. When your complex carbohydrate intake is high and animal protein intake is low to moderate, your body uses the protein more efficiently. The carbohydrates also help keep nitrogen levels high and assist your body's utilization of amino acids in building protein.

If your animal protein intake exceeds the percentage I recommend, your body will likely absorb very little of it and then react as if it were in a protein-starvation situation—which results in nitrogen depletion, poor gains, poor performance, and muscle breakdown. Recent research suggests that athletes have higher protein requirements than the current standard. However, research indicates that consuming more than one gram of protein per pound of lean body weight (excluding the pounds of body fat) can lead to kidney and organ toxicity.

To reiterate an important point, your amino acid supplementation program should be supervised by a professional who is knowledgeable in nutrition and amino acid biochemistry. Keep that in mind if amino acid supplementation becomes part of your Ultimate Sports Nutrition program.

66

11
BRANCHED-CHAIN AMINO ACIDS

As we've seen, you the athlete have a higher protein requirement than other people. But that need presents you with a nutritional dilemma.

You need more protein, but you can pay a high price for it. High protein intake exerts a metabolic toll on your body in the form of extra work for your liver and kidneys, as well as increased losses of water and calcium.

Is there a way for you to meet your high protein needs without the negative consequences associated with protein metabolism? There may be, by concentrating on certain amino acids known as *branched-chain amino acids*, or *BCAAs*.

These three amino acids—leucine, isoleucine, and valine—are called *branched-chain* because of their molecular structure: an amino group (NH_3) on one end and an acid group (COOH) on the other, with various side chains attached to this basic configuration. (Leucine, isoleucine, and valine, incidentally, are essential amino acids; they cannot be made in the body and must be supplied by foods or supplements.)

The tissue-sparing capacities of BCAAs were illustrated in an experiment using infected monkeys. Fed solutions of BCAAs intravenously with other nutrients, the monkeys did not experience the tissue wasting that normally would occur with infection. But other amino acids failed to halt the loss of protein tissue. It's because of these experiments that BCAAs were eventually used to prevent tissue wasting in cancer therapy.

For the athlete, BCAAs present an even more promising characteristic. They can be used as an ergogenic aid—that is, to assist in better physical performance. In fact, these three BCAAs are similar to anabolic steroids in their effects on athletic performance, but they have none of the side effects associated with steroids. Besides their tissue-sparing qualities, they have potent anabolic (building) qualities, and they yield metabolic by-products that boost your energy production for long-term sports activities.

How BCAAs Work in Your Body

When you eat a high-protein meal, the most rapidly absorbed amino acids are the BCAAs. Of all the amino acids processed by your liver, 70 percent of those released into the bloodstream are BCAAs.

The BCAAs are then picked up by your muscle tissues very quickly. In the first three hours after a meal, BCAAs account for 50 to 90 percent of total amino acid uptake by the muscles. Your muscles, in other words, are hungry for these three amino acids in particular.

In fact, your muscles are so greedy for BCAAs that they sometimes absorb too much. That causes the BCAAs to assist your muscles in synthesizing other amino acids needed for the building—that is, anabolic—process. That's pretty much what anabolic steroids do, the difference being, of course, that BCAAs act in a safer way.

Another way BCAAs act—especially leucine—as an ergogenic aid is by stimulating the production of insulin. That means more circulating blood sugar (glucose) will be taken up by the muscle cells and used as an energy source. Insulin acts in concert with BCAAs to drive into the muscle all other amino acids (except for tryptophan) to be used to build muscle tissue.

Branched-chain amino acids differ from the other amino acids in that they're metabolized in the muscle rather than in the liver. That accounts for their rapid uptake by the muscle.

How To Use BCAAs

The three branched-chain amino acids—leucine, isoleucine, and valine—must be available at the same time in order to ensure maximum absorption into the body. In fact, studies indicate that leucine, taken by itself, will actually impair the overall utilization of dietary protein. Adding its partners, isoleucine and valine, however, will offset this negative effect.

If you decide to take BCAA supplements as part of your Ultimate Sports Nutrition diet and to enhance your athletic performance, you have to keep in mind that they actively compete with two other amino acids—tryptophan and tyrosine—for absorption. Since, as we've seen, BCAAs are especially rapidly absorbed, they usually beat out their competition for absorption.

That isn't entirely good, because tryptophan and tyrosine are extremely important for proper brain functioning. Also, tryptophan is a popular remedy for insomnia, pain, and depression. With BCAAs blocking the uptake of these two amino acids, their beneficial effect is nullified.

Solution to the problem? Simply take your BCAAs at different times than you take tryptophan and tyrosine.

If you want to use BCAAs to promote long-term energy benefits, take them no more than 30 minutes before a long-distance event. Because of their insulin-promoting effects, BCAAs can cause some individuals to become particularly sensitive to the drop in blood sugar levels that accompanies the release of insulin. That can lead to the opposite of what you want—premature exhaustion of glycogen stores, resulting in decreased performance.

In order to utilize BCAAs best for enhancing tissue anabolism, consume them within 60 to 90 minutes after a workout. This is the peak time period for amino acid uptake by the muscles. Take one to four grams of each of the three BCAAs.

Remember that all three BCAAs must be present at the same time to do any good. And make sure you're getting enough vitamin B_6— about 50 to 100 milligrams daily—to spark many of the metabolic conversions involving BCAAs.

Clearly, branched-chain amino acids have a place in your supply of ergogenic aids. They stimulate two of the most desired effects in sports performance: energy production for muscular work and anabolic processes within the muscle cells.

12
CAFFEINE

There is no doubt about the efficacy of caffeine in aiding sports performance. Caffeine works. It is known to stimulate the central nervous system, mobilize various hormones and tissue substrates that are involved in metabolic processes, improve muscle contraction, and improve the mobilization and utilization rates of fats and carbohydrates for energy.

But—and this is a big *but*—*how* you use caffeine is of critical importance in whether it will yield maximum performance benefits for you. Here are some important points to consider:

- Explosive-power athletes—those who do short-duration sports such as lifting, sprints, etc.—appear not to benefit from caffeine use.
- Endurance athletes—long-distance cyclists, runners, swimmers, etc.—can improve their performance with caffeine use.
- Reaction time can be improved with caffeine.
- Heavy coffee drinkers (two to six cups per day) will, upon forced abstinence, experience increased reaction time when they "go back on."
- Administering caffeine to heavy users decreases their reaction time and relieves anxiety.

- The best dose is about three milligrams of caffeine per kilogram of body weight. Below that, little performance improvement is noted, and above that, there will be a performance decrement.
- Administering caffeine to an athlete who uses less than two cups of coffee daily, and who has abstained from it for several days results in improved performance.
- Improved uptake of free fatty acids by the muscle cells and enhanced use of muscle triglycerides are responsible for improved performance in endurance sports. Both are facilitated by caffeine ingestion. The net effect of the above two functions is that an overall glycogen-sparing process occurs, a plus for long endurance sports such as the marathon or triathlon.
- Fat loss with exercise is increased when caffeine 2.5 to 3.0 milligrams per kilogram body weight is taken prior to exercise.
- The half-life of caffeine in your blood is about 2 to 2½ hours. Its ergogenic effects therefore are of similar duration.
- Because caffeine penetrates the blood-brain barrier, it exerts a powerful influence upon the sensorimotor cortex of the brain. This results in increased alertness, reduced drowsiness, and a reduced perception of fatigue.

With the above considerations in mind, it would seem beneficial to use caffeine before training or competition in most sports—even those requiring power, strength, or skill. Endurance capabilities seem most responsive to caffeine use, but other athletes may benefit from the improved alertness and reaction time (contractility). This may be especially true for athletes such as powerlifters, weightlifters, wrestlers, and decathletes, who engage in multiple bouts throughout an extended period of time.

Again, however, not everyone responds well to caffeine ingestion. Costill noted that about 20 percent of the population will exhibit enough adverse effects from caffeine to preclude its use as an ergogenic aid. DeVries (1974) found that caffeine can negatively affect carbohydrate and protein metabolism. Other adverse effects of caffeine include cardiac arrhythmias, excessive diuresis (urination), insomnia, withdrawal headaches, and types of anxiety indistinguishable from anxiety neurosis called *caffeinism*. If you're among the 20 percent who cannot tolerate caffeine, forget about it. The small kick you get from it isn't worth the side effects.

People with ulcers also are cautioned against using caffeine because it causes a 400 percent increase in acid levels in the gut.

As mentioned above, the best dose for improved performance is about three milligrams of caffeine per kilogram (2.2 pounds) of body weight. Taken in the form of coffee, this translates to about two cups of black coffee ingested one hour before the athletic event. However, remember that the most effective dosage varies considerably from athlete to athlete. Also keep in mind that you're using caffeine as an ergogenic aid, not as part of your Ultimate Sports Nutrition program, since caffeine has no nutritive value.

A final note on taking caffeine as a supplement: Don't take it with niacin, because niacin has the opposite effect on fat metabolism. Niacin blocks fatty acid release from fat cells, though niacinamide doesn't have this effect.

13
D,L,PHENYLALANINE (DLPA)

Athletes learn to live with pain. Some accept it as a way of life—the price of glory. I don't like pain, and I try my best to get rid of it. Most often I succeed. But many athletes suffer from chronic pain from such ailments as joint inflammation, torn or strained muscles or tendons, migraines, and arthritis.

Chronic pain is tough to take and is almost always debilitating in sports performance. One treatment that many athletes find successful is nutritional control of pain with one of the eight essential amino acids, phenylalanine. Specifically, they supplement their diet with tablets containing a special form of phenylalanine commonly abbreviated as *DLPA*. This substance comes in three forms: d, l, and a mixture of equal parts of d and l. (Your body converts the d type to the l type for utilization.)

DLPA works by intensifying and prolonging your body's own natural painkilling response. The brain responds to painkilling signals by producing hormones called *endorphins*, which have properties similar to those of morphine, a powerful analgesic drug. But enzymes in the body tend to destroy much of the endorphins, and injecting them into the body has proved infeasible.

Researchers have discovered that d and d,l,phenylalanine inhibit these enzymes from destroying the endorphins, giving them a longer life span in which to exert their powerful pain-relieving actions.

So, *supplementing the diet with DLPA allows the brain to act normally in its reaction to pain signals and then allows the reaction to continue for a much longer period by protecting endorphin hormones from enzymatic inactivation. So the pain-relieving actions of DLPA occur through natural means, in contrast to drugs.*

It is important to follow the proper dosage schedule for best results with DLPA. Start with two tablets of 375 milligrams of DLPA taken 15 to 30 minutes before each meal, for a total of six tablets daily. Continue until you experience a substantial relief in pain— usually within four days, but sometimes in two or three weeks— then double the initial dosage for another two to three weeks. If this doesn't work, discontinue use. Only 5 to 15 percent of users don't get relief from DLPA.

DLPA may be used along with other analgesics, such as aspirin-type compounds. Also, common antiarthritic drugs such as Indocin, Motrin, and Naprosyn are compatible with DLPA and can increase its effectiveness.

DLPA is not intended for use by phenylketonurics or during pregnancy. Persons with high blood pressure should take DLPA after meals.

14
BEE POLLEN

Somewhere along the way, a myth evolved that bee pollen is a superfood endowing its users with amazing health and physical prowess. According to Tim Larkin, writing for *Consumer*, published by the Department of Health and Human Services, there is no valid scientific evidence of any therapeutic benefit from bee pollen.

I don't recommend that you include bee pollen as part of your Ultimate Sports Nutrition program or as an ergogenic aid. Why not? Because it's useless.

Bee pollen is legally marketed as a food, but not as a drug. "If those selling bee pollen . . . claim it can cure or alleviate any illness or produce some therapeutic benefit, the law says the product is a drug and must meet rigid scientific requirements for both safety and effectiveness," Larkin says. "Obviously, some bee pollen distributors have been making drug claims."

The FDA has shut down this practice by asking bee pollen manufacturers to recall their product and promotional literature. The FDA also has powers of seizure, injunction, and criminal prosecution when an unapproved drug or product is classified as a drug due to the therapeutic claims made for it.

Here are some of the claims made for bee pollen and the facts about it:

1. *Bee pollen improves athletic performance:* Untrue. A 1975 study by the National Association of Athletic Trainers tested a

swim team in which half took 10 bee pollen tablets a day for six months. One-quarter took 10 placebo tablets, and the other one-quarter received 5 pollen and 5 placebo tablets. There was no measurable difference in performance among the three groups. A later test with swimmers and runners led researchers to conclude that bee pollen was "absolutely not a significant aid in metabolism, workout training or performance."

2. *Pollen is a giant germ killer in which bacteria cannot exist.* Nonsense. When exposed to air, pollen is rapidly attacked by bacteria, yeast, and other fungi.

3. *Pollen is nature's most perfect food.* In fact, it is the best food *only for bees.*

4. *Pollen retards aging, as evidenced by the longevity of natives of Russia's Georgian mountains, who owe it all to their pollen-rich diet.* Actually, these hardy folks happen to eat a Pritikin-type diet with about 70 percent of calories obtained from vegetables. They eat honey, but they made no mention of bee pollen when talking to researchers.

5. *Pollen is the richest source of protein known to science.* Wrong again. Actually, the major component of pollen is carbohydrate. Protein content varies from 5 to 28 percent, depending on the plant from which it comes. By comparison, tofu contains 46 percent protein; raw soybeans, 38 percent; dry pumpkin seed, 29 percent; brewer's yeast, 39 percent; and round steak, 20 percent.

6. *Bee pollen relieves allergies, asthma, and hay fever.* There are no scientific studies to support this claim. On the contrary, scientists believe that bee pollen is especially hazardous for persons with allergies, asthma, or hay fever.

Some people believe bee pollen contains a special substance that science hasn't yet identified. This may be, but until the supposedly magic ingredient comes to light, be wary of false advertising claims. There are other ergogenic aids more deserving of your attention, ingestion, and investment than bee pollen.

15
L-CARNITINE

Most people probably have never heard of L-carnitine. But Dr. Guillermo Laich of Madrid, Spain, one of the world's foremost experts in sports medicine and human performance, suggests that L-carnitine, because of its unique biological properties, may play an important role in endurance athletic events. He further states that L-carnitine is absolutely essential in cellular fat transport.

How can this mysterious substance, familiar only to biochemists, improve sports performance as part of your Ultimate Sports Nutrition program?

L-carnitine, discovered in meat extracts in 1905 by Russian scientists, was named after the Latin word *carnis*, which means "meat" or "flesh." Scientists working with liver cells note that carnitine seemed to act as a fat carrier, allowing fat to be transported into the mitochrondia of cells, where it's used as energy.

This discovery has tremendous implications for athletes because it seems to indicate that L-carnitine accelerates the fat-oxidation, or fat-burning, process. This would lead to lower body fat as well as increased long-term energy for more intense workouts.

In addition, L-carnitine stimulates the burning of the amino acids leucine and valine, which contribute up to 10 percent of energy production during intense exercise. Thus, carnitine may assist in maintaining normal energy output during periods of fasting or reduced intake of fat or carbohydrates, as occurs during strict dieting.

One problem with certain diets involves ketosis, the overproduction of ketones, which is the by-product of incomplete combustion of fat. Ketosis is common during diets extremely low in carbohydrates or calories. Large amounts of ketones can be toxic to the brain and nervous system, leading to dehydration as the body attempts to eliminate them through the kidneys. This diuretic effect results in the loss of valuable electrolytes, such as potassium, causing extreme weakness and fatigue.

Working with rats, Dr. Y. Yeh reported in a 1981 issue of *Journal of Nutrition* that L-carnitine has an antiketogenic effect. If this is confirmed in humans, L-carnitine may help minimize the negative effects of fat burning associated with dieting.

L-carnitine can be obtained from muscle meats and animal protein foods and can be synthesized from two amino acids, lysine and methionine. The natural L-carnitine content of some selected foods is shown in the accompanying table.

Carnitine Content of Selected Foods (in mg per 100 g)

Sheep (muscle)	210.0
Lamb (muscle)	78.0
Beef (muscle)	64.0
Chicken (muscle)	7.5
Lamb (liver)	2.6
Yeast	2.4
Cow's milk	2.0

L-carnitine is virtually nonexistent in vegetables and fruits, and most strict vegetarian diets are low in the L-carnitine building blocks of lysine and methionine. Vegetarians risk L-carnitine deficiency unless the missing nutrients are supplemented in the diet. This possibly explains why most bodybuilders who go on a strict vegetarian diet notice an immediate loss of strength and muscle function. (The lack of vitamin B_{12} in these diets also may be a factor).

In order for L-carnitine to be synthesized in the body, a few accessory nutrients that act as coenzymes or catalysts must be present. Besides the amino acids lysine and methionine, this process requires vitamins C, B_6, and niacin, as well as iron.

As with amino acids, carnitine is found in two basic forms, L-carnitine and D-carnitine. Thus far, the only toxic effect noticed with the L form has been a transient diarrhea, which occurred when huge doses (more than 10 grams) were given.

However, the D-form can be toxic to the body by blocking the function of the more useful L form. This can lead to severe muscle weakness. D-carnitine also inhibits the enzymes that allow L-carnitine to transport fat into the cell, thus inhibiting the fat-burning process.

Some health food stores are selling a carnitine product that combines the D and L forms. Because of the toxicity factors associated with the D-form it's best to avoid this type of product.

L-carnitine may be valuable in treating certain heart diseases, particularly hardening of the arteries. In Europe, doctors prescribe L-carnitine for this purpose. By promoting maximal cellular uptake of fats, L-carnitine may ease the work load of the heart, which prefers the fuel supplied by fatty acids. A large amount of fatty acids at one time, though, can precipitate a fatal heart rhythm disturbance called *ventricular arrhythmia*. By helping transport fats into the cells, L-carnitine may help prevent this type of irregularity.

It's apparent that L-carnitine may enhance several physiological functions relevant to athletes. It plays an essential role in transport of fat into the cells, where it is burned as energy. By promoting maximal cellular uptake of fat, L-carnitine can improve fat metabolism and possibly aid in lowering body fat levels. It also may allow a more efficient processing of fat, leading to increased energy levels for long-term activities, such as aerobic exercise and long weight-training sessions. And, coupled with other nutrients, L-carnitine may spare dieters some of the unpleasant side effects of restricted food intake, such as ketosis.

Unfortunately, L-carnitine, the most biologically active form of this nutrient, currently is available in only prohibitively expensive forms. But don't despair! Even though it's available as a supplement, the safest way, currently, to add more of this valuable substance to your system may be to allow the natural processes of your body to take over and produce it for you. Since the major portion of L-carnitine can be biosynthesized from other building-block nutrients, you can increase your body's supply of carnitine by ingesting generous amounts of the amino acids lysine and methionine, bolstered by iron and vitamins C and B_6. This shouldn't be difficult, as long as your diet includes meals (refer back to the list of carnitine-rich foods) that supply the necessary raw materials.

16
INOSINE

You shouldn't think of ergogenic aids as substitutes for the sound nutrition principles that you're applying to your Ultimate Sports Nutrition program. But the advantages that inosine has to offer in improving your workouts are too great to be ignored. It's a safe, legal, and effective supplement.

All the mental discipline in the world, all the guts and determination, simply aren't capable of helping you force out that last muscle-building rep if there's no more ATP in your muscle cells. ATP (adenosine triphosphate) is the chemical in your body that allows your muscles to contract. It's the only substance that can do this. When your workout is fast and furious, your muscles can't replace ATP quickly enough. The result is fatigued muscles.

If only you could replace ATP quickly, think of the energy you'd have. You'd get that last rep, and perhaps a couple more to boot. And soon, over weeks, those extra reps would add up to improved strength from the more intense overload.

Athletes the world over are now falling over one another to procure a substance that can do just that. It's called *inosine*, and it's available in the United States in health food stores.

My first exposure to inosine came in 1983, when I was in Moscow studying at the Institute of Sport. I befriended some of the weight-lifters there and was given some to take back home with me. I found that it provided an energy boost to my training of a magnitude I'd never experienced.

Japanese researchers discovered inosine while searching for a substitute for the cardiac stimulant digitalis. Heart patients suffering from an irregular heartbeat or angina benefit from digitalis's action in promoting continued smooth cardiac operation. Inosine has the same effect, the Japanese found.

Inosine belongs to a chemical family known as *purine nucleotides*. It easily penetrates cell walls of both cardiac and skeletal muscle. Once inside, it promotes the manufacture of more ATP. It also promotes the production of another biochemical called *2,3,diphosphoglycerate (2,3,DPG)*. This substance is essential for facilitating the transport of oxygen molecules from the red blood cells to the muscle cell for energy.

The Japanese touted their discovery as helpful in the treatment of acute and chronic myocarditis, myocardiosclerosis, senile heart, myocardial infarction, and heart arrhythmia. For athletes, though, anecdotal evidence suggests that inosine may be helpful in metabolizing sugar and thereby improving metabolism and ATP production, improving the respiratory process, synthesizing protein, and promoting oxygen transport. All of these benefits aid athletes by improving their energy levels during periods of extreme fatigue.

Many athletes, including powerlifters, have found that over-the-counter inosine tablets help them achieve levels of strength (from improved training over time) that rival the effectiveness of anabolic steriods. Inosine acts on a short-term basis and can be taken every day. The recommended dosage is approximately 1,000 to 1,200 milligrams just before your workout.

While the Japanese researchers caution against the use of inosine if you suffer from gout—excess uric acid in the blood, causing swelling and pain in the joints—it appears to be free of any noticeable ill effects for otherwise healthy athletes.

In my book, it's about time something came along that appears to be safe, yet delivers the boost all athletes demand. At the very least, inosine is a step in the right direction. Perhaps someday soon, anabolic steroids will be a thing of the past.

17
BLOOD BUFFERS

All athletes who have experienced the debilitating effects of lactic acid buildup will be glad to learn about blood buffers. The accumulation of lactic acid, a by-product of exercise that leaves the muscles sore and tired, may be delayed with the use of sodium phosphate as a blood buffer.

Blood buffers are highly alkaline substances that metabolize lactic acid, thus delaying the onset of muscle fatigue. Recent research shows that sodium phosphate not only decreases blood lactate levels but also elevates oxygen uptake (VO_2 max, the ability of the blood to extract oxygen)—both desirable effects for athletic performance.

One study used 10 trained runners with average pretest VO_2 max levels of 56 milliliters per kilogram per minute. After taking one gram of sodium phosphate four times a day for three days, their blood lactate levels dropped from 5 milliequivalents (a unit of volume measurement) to below 4 milliequivalents.

Sodium phosphate seems to increase levels of 2,3,DPG, which increases oxygen uptake and decreases lactic acid buildup. Ingestion of simple baking soda (sodium bicarbonate) may inhibit lactic acid buildup that interferes with work capacity. The dosage used in research was 300 milligrams per kilogram of body weight. Thus, the recommended dosage for a person weighing 70 kilograms would be about 21 grams. One side effect noted with use of sodium bicarbonate was diarrhea.

People with sodium retention problems or high blood pressure should not use blood buffers. More research is needed in this area, but preliminary investigations suggest that blood buffers may help to improve athletes' performance by delaying onset of fatigue, particularly in untrained individuals.

18
ADENOSINE TRIPHOSPHATE

One of the reasons inosine is such an effective energy booster is that it induces the production of adenosine triphosphate (ATP) in your muscle cells. What would happen if you could consume ATP directly as a supplement? A lot, since ATP powers muscle contractions, ignites nerve tissue, provides the energy for body tissue repair, and fuels the energy transformations involved in reproduction and growth.

"ATP drives the process of life," says Francis J. Carniglia, a veterinarian who has been researching the substance for some 40 years. "It's the fountainhead that fuels the energy needs of man, animals, plants, and one-celled bacteria."

Carniglia has, in fact, developed an ATP nutritional supplement that he has used successfully on race horses. For humans, ATP is now used only for pharmaceutical purposes; it remains for future research to come up with a supplement program designed specifically to increase ATP in human muscle.

ATP is manufactured by a small structure located inside the cell, the mitochondria, called "the powerhouse of the cell." The mitochondria population of a muscle cell has been used as a means of estimating the cell's potential energy supply. The more mitochondria in a muscle cell, the greater its energy potential.

Dr. Carniglia's work is directed toward increasing the levels of

ATP in cell mitochondria. In horses on the special dietary supplement, "it was not unusual to see a doubling of the ATP levels in as short a time as 11 days," said Dr. Carniglia. In some cases, the gains in ATP levels were almost five-fold. The lower the ATP levels prior to dietary enrichment, the greater the increase in ATP values afterward.

The horses also exhibited a sense of well-being, with a noticeable increase in their capacity and willingness to do work, he reported.

"The energy levels of the body can be elevated," says Dr. Carniglia. "This accomplishment has many potential applications from one-celled bacteria to multicelled people and all the species in between."

Research by Tyson and Associates, manufacturers of pharmaceuticals and nutritional supplements, summarized the ATP research by stating that "ATP is of considerable significance to the living organism in numerous ways."

According to Tyson, ATP produces "superior effects" in treating muscular diseases, such as progressive muscular atrophy, myasthenia, and progressive neuralgic amyotrophy, as well as diseases of the heart, brain, skin, ears, and eyes. "ATP is a very safe substance. There is no contraindication except in the case of hypotension," said Tyson.

19
METHYL DONORS: TMG AND DMG

Every athlete has experienced burning, sore muscles, fatigue, and even cramps after a strenuous workout or competition. These conditions are due to the buildup of lactic acid, a by-product of vigorous exercise caused by low oxygenation to the muscles.

Improving oxygen delivery to the muscles has been a goal of sports research scientists, for it would mean improving muscle efficiency and maximizing athletic performance. It appears that this goal has been reached with discovery of how *methyl donors* contribute to a vital biochemical process called *transmethylation*.

Methyl donors are important to oxygenation: the more methyl groups that are available in a nutrient, the more oxygen can be delivered to the muscles.

Methyl donors act as biochemical catalysts to enhance biological efficiency through their many contributions to cellular reactions. Methyl donors are involved in the synthesis of protein and nucleic acid (DNA and RNA) and in maintaining the integrity of the nervous system.

The most familiar methyl donor is dimethylglycine, or DMG, also known as vitamin B_{15}. This substance, which Durk Pearson and Sandy Shaw promote as an immune system stimulant in their best-selling book *Life Extension*, is discussed at the end of this chapter.

Trimethylglycine (TMG)

The latest discovery in boosting oxygen delivery to the muscles is a chemical cousin of DMG—trimethylglycine, or TMG. As the prefix *tri* suggests, this substance contains three methyl groups, making it an even more potent and useful nutrient than DMG.

TMG is a natural metabolite of the body, produced when there are sufficient quantities of its dietary precursors, choline and the essential amino acid methionine. TMG donates its three methyl groups to the vital process of transmethylation, which transforms eight amino acids to more than 100 other specific-function amino acids.

Methyl groups are found naturally in such foods as beef, pork, liver, egg yolk, wheat germ, and peanuts. Some concern has been expressed that the popular low-cholesterol/low-fat diets may lack sufficient methyl groups. People on these diets should take supplements containing methyl groups.

TMG supplements, such as glycine betaine, are derived from beets. The parent compound, betaine, is available as a compound with hydrochloric acid for use as a digestive aid. However, this form is far too caustic to be considered for use as an athletic performance booster.

A recommended form is TMG tablets, available in 100 milligram potency. Take one to three tablets daily (100 to 300 milligrams) to increase athletic stamina and endurance. If you can't find TMG supplements, don't despair—substitute choline, which also supplies three methyl groups. Choline is manufactured in the body from the amino acids methionine or serine.

Dimethylglycine (DMG)

Although not as potent an oxygenation enhancer, DMG is a substance many athletes use and swear by.

DMG has been referred to as the "Russian vitamin." Since the mid-sixties, a staggering amount of research has come out of the Soviet Union concerning the oxygenating effects of DMG. A growing number of physicians who now routinely prescribe DMG (average dose, 60 milligrams per day) for their heart patients are reporting generally favorable responses.

Incidentally, the Soviets used calcium pangamate, or pangamic acid, as their DMG source. To date, I have noticed no real differences in reported efficacies of DMG (believed to be the active ingredient in calcium pangamate) and calcium pangamate. DMG is typically taken sublingually (under the tongue), while the "Russian" formula is taken in pill form.

Since no deficiency state has been noted for this substance, the FDA does not classify it as a vitamin. Further, several studies have found no significant inprovement in performance capabilities among athletes using DMG, giving rise to an array of academic disbelievers. But to athletes—growing numbers of them—who use DMG, it's accepted as a substance that delivers.

20
HERBS

Flowers to relieve sore muscles? Potatoes to heal a bruise? Lemons and berries as pain relievers? What goes on?

Some ergogenic aids—any natural substances that enhance athletic performance—are actually traditional, age-old medicines and remedies supplied by the original caretaker and good doctor, Mother Earth. In our high-tech world of synthetic drugs and artificial cures, we sometimes forget the wealth of wonderful substances we can find right under our noses.

What did people do before modern medicine? They found that the Earth is truly a great provider of all man's needs, including medical ones. Common plants were found to contain not only natural remedies but also boosters that, even today, assist us in our quest for optimal sports performance.

Eleutherococcus: The Soviet Superdrug

Eleutherococcus (EC) is derived from the Aaliaceae family of shrubs—a "cousin" of ginseng, with which it often is confused. It has been used extensively in the Soviet Union for more than two decades but is virtually unknown in Western pharmacology. Soviet athletes swear by the stuff. What do they know about it that we don't?

In sports, EC has been found to increase stamina and endurance with no discernible negative side effects.

In one Soviet study, runners participating in a 10-mile race were given EC before the race, while the control group were administered an inactive placebo substance. The athletes in the EC group chopped a whopping five minutes off the finishing time as compared to the placebo group!

94

In a series of experiments conducted at the prestigious Lesgraft Institute of Physical Culture and Sport in Moscow, Professor Igor Korobkov gave EC to 1,500 athletes. Results indicated that EC increased endurance, reflexes, and concentration, particularly in the longer endurance events. EC also appeared to increase the training recovery ability of athletes. The only side effect noticed was a mild, transient increase in blood pressure in some of the athletes.

Professor Korobkov believes that EC should not be included on "doping lists" of banned substances because its action is of a restorative nature rather than that of a drug-induced performance booster. Doping substances are taken with the goal of increasing athletic performance, but EC is used as a year-round health tonic to combat the effects of stress on the body.

Professor Korobkov's argument is rather moot, however, since Western scientists have expressed no interest in banning EC in athletic competition. Western scientists just don't believe in the stuff, so they have no reason to ban it.

Their Soviet counterparts fully believe that EC possesses unique tonic effects. They use it in the treatment of anemia, depression, and heart and blood vessel surgery. The Soviets use it not as a cure, but rather as what they call a "restorative," which they believe acts as an antistress agent.

Soviet scientists first took note of EC as an ergogenic aid while studying its effects on mice. In stress tests, the mice were forced to swim to exhaustion. The rodents that took EC were able to prolong their swimming time by 44 percent. Subsequent human testing showed that EC improved stamina, motivation, coordination, and concentration.

The active compounds in EC and ginseng turned out to be chemicals bound to sugars called *glycosides*. The glycosides in ginseng have chemical structures similar to those of steroid compounds, which partially explains some of the toxic effects noted with a large intake of ginseng, the "ginseng abuse syndrome." The glycosides found in EC are far less toxic than the ginseng variety.

These glycosides are active compounds capable of stimulating the brain but causing none of the side effects noted with drugs such as amphetamines. The glycosides are hypothesized to be active in an area of the brain that initiates the stress response of the body. EC stimulates secretion of these stress-altering chemicals, producing a restorative effect.

While Western scientists cast wary eyes at cure-alls, Soviet research points to substances such as EC as possessing potent normalizing and sustaining effects on many bodily systems. The Western skepticism is ironic, for Westerners readily recognize the negative effects of uncontrolled stress, yet they refuse to accept the possibility of modulating these stress effects through a central brain mechanism stimulated by a safe, natural substance such as EC.

It cannot be denied, however, that the Soviets have superior performance records in many sports events, especially those requiring raw power and stamina. This points to the necessity of keeping an open mind when considering the value of esoteric substances such as EC to promote athletic recovery.

Perhaps someday an iconoclastic Western scientist will be willing to step forward amid the skepticism of his peers and perform the necessary controlled experiments to determine the true value to human performance of substances such as EC and ginseng.

Ginseng

This Chinese perennial herb with an aromatic root has been revered in Far Eastern countries for centuries because of its alleged curative powers.

The Soviets have been particularly effusive in their praise of ginseng's "medicinal properties." For example, Dr. Ivan Brekham of the U.S.S.R. says that "daily doses of ginseng for 15–45 days increase physical endurance and mental work capacity."

Another researcher, Dr. Stephen Dulder, an American, discovered that ginseng works by increasing the efficiency of the adrenal and pituitary glands.

Soviet scientists refer to ginseng as an *adaptogen*, which increases muscle endurance and relieves stress. Substances in ginseng know as *ginsenosides* have a strong chemical structure similar to adrenal steroids and may be responsible for ginseng's reputation as an ergogenic aid and rejuvenator.

Although ginseng is a natural herb, overuse of this substance can lead to what Dr. Ronald Siegal of U.C.L.A. dubs *ginseng abuse syndrome,* or *G.A.S.:* insomnia, nervousness, irritability, high blood pressure, diarrhea, and skin manifestations such as rashes and swelling.

In addition, women are cautioned that estrogenlike compounds found in ginseng can cause breast tenderness, vaginal bleeding, and menstrual irregularities.

When taken in moderation in the form of mild tea, ginseng appears to be a safe, mild stimulant. However, excess amounts should be avoided to prevent the G.A.S. syndrome.

96

Herbs for Athletic Injuries

Here are a few simple herbal remedies for common athletic injuries, such as twisting the ankle, knee, or shoulder. Most of these remedies will help reduce swelling and inflammation and ease the pain—and they should be used with the standard RICE first-aid treatment (rest, ice, compression, and elevation).

Serious injuries, of course, require a physician's care.

Arnica Compress

This longtime remedy, said to speed healing of bruises, strains, and sprains, consists of one tablespoon of arnica tincture *(Tinctura Arnica)* in one pint of cold water. Wet a towel with the mixture and apply it to the injured area.

You can purchase arnica tincture (often called arnica "extract") at a pharmacy. Or make your own by soaking a handful of fresh arnica flowers in one pint of ethyl alcohol (70 percent) for two weeks.

Marigold

This common flower *(Calendula officinalis)* provides several remedies that relieve muscle soreness from exercise. No medicine cabinet should be without marigold tincture and salve.

Bath additive: Add two handsful of fresh marigold (flowers and leaves) or three ounces of dried marigold to one or two quarts of hot water. Steep for 20 minutes, strain, and add the liquid to the bath water. Wrap the strained herb in a linen sack and put it into the bath.

Tincture: Soak a handful of flowers in one quart of brandy. Store in the sun or a warm place for two weeks. Strain. To use, dilute with distilled water.

Salve: Mix one to two teaspoons of fresh marigold juice with one ounce of lard. Or add two handsful of fresh, cut flowers and leaves to one-half pound of hot lard. Mix, remove from heat, and let stand overnight. Heat again, strain, and store in a jar.

Other Bath Additives

To relax tense, overworked muscles and relieve the worst of pain, soak in a hot bath with special additives of juniper *(Juniperus cummuunis* or *J. oxycedrus)* berries or young twigs of lemon balm *(Melissa officinalis).*

Remedy for Bruises

Freshly grate a raw potato, apply it to the bruised area, and leave it on for 15 minutes or as long as it feels comfortable. Potatoes are the richest natural source of potassium chloride, the most effective of all potassium compounds when it comes to healing bruises.

Low Back Pain

Many athletes and dancers are afflicted with low back pain, the result of injury, inherent weakness, or simple abuse. There are two herbal remedies that help ease chronic back pain: hot linseed poultice and massage with Saint-John's-wort oil. (Note: Acute pain should never be treated with heat. Apply ice and seek professional help.)

Linseed poultice: Soak one cup of linseeds in cold water overnight. Bring to a boil and apply as hot as is tolerable. Can be reheated a few times.

Saint-John's-wort massage: Add fresh Saint-John's-wort flowers *(Hypericum perforatum)* to a jar and cover with olive oil. Tightly close the jar and store in a warm place or in the sun for three to five weeks (the oil will turn red). Strain. Pour the oil into a dark-colored glass jar and store in a dark, cool area. Don't refrigerate.

Comfrey

Folk healers used this favorite remedy for all sorts of athletic injuries, including damaged cartilage, musculoskeletal injuries, and generally speeding up the healing process.

Comfrey tea: Add two teaspoons of cut comfrey rootstock to one cup of cold water and soak overnight. Or add one teaspoon of cut comfrey leaves to one cup of hot water and steep for five minutes. Strain. Drink two to four cups throughout the day.

Comfrey poultice: Add hot water and a few drops of olive oil to dried, chopped comfrey rootstock or rootstock powder until a thick mash is formed. Spread on linen cloth and apply to the injured area. Renew every two to four hours.

98

Antispasmodic Tea

This brew helps relieve and prevent muscle cramps and spasms. Mix one ounce of chamomile flowers *(Maricaria chamomilla)*, cinquefoil *(Potenitalla anserina)*, lemon balm *(Melissa officinalis)*, and hops *(Mumulus lupulus)* and one-half ounce of valcrian *(Valeriana officinalis)*. Add one teaspoon of the herbal mixture to one cup of hot water, steep for three minutes, strain and drink.

Chinese Herbs

In recent years the Western world has expressed renewed interest in traditional Chinese medicine, including herbal remedies. Among the Chinese herbs useful to athletes are Ma Huang *(Ephedra sinica)*, Fo-ti-tieng *(Polygonum multiflorum)*, and *Radix astregulus*. These herbs traditionally were used to integrate one's physical and mental powers, or *chi*. They originally were used in meditation centers to increase attention and mental clarity.

Specifically, here's what these ingredients are said to do:

Ma Huang (Ephedra sinica)

This herb contains 19 or more major active ingredients, one of which provides the basis for synthetic ephedrine. Ma Huang has warming properties, stimulating the cerebral cortex while increasing heart rate. The bronchi of the lungs are relaxed and dilated, easing breathing. Ma Huang has diaphoretic, diuretic, and decongestant properties. Ma Huang's principal action is to break up stoppage in the chi flow.

Fo-ti-tieng (Polygonum multiflorum)

This herb is believed to possess remarkable rejuvenating properties. Appearing often in Chinese prescriptions for regeneration, it is reputed to enhance memory, decrease fatigue, nourish the blood, strengthen bones and tendons, and calm nerves.

Radix Astregulus

This herb is favored in China as a tonic and diuretic. It is a specific tonic to the "triple heater," the Oriental concept for the main energy flow of the lungs (breathing), intestines (digestion), and elimination (regeneration). Radix astregulus is considered good nourishment for smooth muscles and skin. It strengthens energies and aids tissue regeneration.

One U.S. company markets a product called Chi Power made from these Chinese herbs in capsule form. The manufacturers say "Chi Power" will brighten mental awareness and stimulate physical processes while not causing the nervousness associated with caffeine. Some professional and amateur athletes have found this product useful in focusing energies and improving respiration.

21
SUPERCHARGED HEMOGLOBIN

Mention "blood doping" to the man in the street, and he'll probably think of a room full of strung-out junkies anxiously awaiting their next fix.

Athletes know that in reality blood doping doesn't involve any kind of dope. What it does involve is simply the extraction, followed by a later reinfusion, of an athlete's blood to improve sports performance.

The efficacy of the technique was evident at the 1984 Summer Olympic Games. Some U.S. cyclists left their competitors wondering if the U.S. had come up with invisible motors for their bikes. It was later revealed that these athletes had employed blood doping under the careful supervision of several prominent team physicians.

The blood doping technique is simple. About a pint of blood is removed from the athlete and stored (frozen) for three to four weeks or more. In the meantime, the athlete's body compensates for the loss by manufacturing additional red blood cells. Red cells contain a protein-iron pigment called *hemoglobin*, which locks on to oxygen molecules and carries them via the bloodstream to all the cells in the body. The blood is then thawed and reinfused two to three days before the competition, adding to the total number of oxygen-carrying red blood cells.

Oxygen's Role in Athletic Performance

Oxygen is responsible for sparking many energy processes necessary for life. An increase in hemoglobin means increased capacity for oxygen transport to the muscles, which means an increase in endurance.

Scientists have been experimenting with raising the hemoglobin content of blood ever since they theorized that athletes training in the thin oxygen of high altitudes would compensate by producing extra hemoglobin. Current research, however, contradicts this theory. It is now believed that high-altitude training causes a *decrease*, not an increase, in the concentration of plasma (the liquid part of blood). This dehydration effect creates thicker blood and is believed to be detrimental to athletic performance.

So the scientists set to work on blood-doping techniques. After the method was refined, long-distance track records fell with each international meet. Finland's Lass Viren, for example, would finish a grueling 10,000-meter run looking like he could do it all over again. But when asked the secret of his superlative performance, Viren shrugged and replied, "Bee pollen." Viren was not yet ready to divulge the full extent of his Draculean experimentation.

There are currently proposed bans on blood doping in athletic competition. Banning blood doping isn't a bad idea, because it's a risky practice. One risk is that of infection from using dirty needles. Another significant problem in this system is storage. Poor storage techniques can destroy the key chemical in the process, 2,3, Diphosphoglycerate—2,3, DPG for short. The fragile 2,3, DPG is the element in the hemoglobin molecule that binds to, and then releases, oxygen for availability to the cells. When 2,3, DPG disappears, the efficacy of the doping method drops.

Phytic Acid

An advancement in the blood-doping method recently was made when scientists isolated the part of hemoglobin where 2,3, DPG binds into oxygen. To increase the oxygen delivery capacity of hemoglobin, they now use an analog or chemical cousin of 2,3, DPG called *phytic acid.* Substituting phytic acid for 2,3, DPG produces a looser bind to oxygen. This loose binding permits about twice as much oxygen per unit of blood to be delivered to the tissues.

Increased oxygen delivery relieves strain from the heart, whose main job is to pump oxygen-laden blood to the body's tissues.

Research is now under way to apply this new oxygenation technique to a medical condition called *ischemia*, or lack of blood flow to a specific area of the body. Scientists are operating on the premise that any tissue kept supplied with oxygen has a greater chance of living or working properly.

To incorporate phytic acid into red blood cells, the researchers first bathe the cells in a solution of DMSO (dimethyl sulfoxide), which has a small molecule that easily penetrates the cells. Once inside the cells, the solution is diluted, causing the red blood cells to swell. The bathing solution also contains phytic acid, which can penetrate the cell membranes only when the cells are swollen. As phytic acid enters the cells, the DMSO is forced out and the cell shrinks back to its normal size, trapping the phytic acid inside.

The result: supercharged hemoglobin—and vastly increased oxygen delivery to the cells.

Pyridoxine

There's another, even more potent technique for improving blood oxygenation: using a derivative of vitamin B_6, or pyridoxine, instead of phytic acid.

When locked on to hemoglobin, pyridoxine acts as a super DPG. It's 10 times as effective as 2,3, DPG in making oxygen available to the cells.

Supercharging the hemoglobin with such a potent substance has valuable medical applications. It prevents the hemoglobin from splitting after delivering oxygen to the system, thus delaying the excretion of hemoglobin through the kidneys. This prolongs the oxygen-delivering capacity of hemoglobin.

Also, unlike "normal" hemoglobin, "supercharged" hemoglobin can deliver oxygen at very low temperatures. This makes it ideal for transporting organs for surgical transplant procedures. The supercharged hemoglobin allows the organs to be stored at very low temperatures to preserve cell structure and supplies the oxygen required to keep these cells functional.

With the proposed bans on blood doping in athletic competition, you can bet that sooner or later a sports scientist will modify these new techniques for use by athletes. So watch out—when this happens, you'll see some significant changes in the record books!

22
GAMA-ORYZANOL

As an athlete, you've probably been exposed to a wide variety of ergogenic aids—some effective and some ineffective, some safe and some risky, some organic and some manmade. Undoubtedly you'd jump at the chance to find one that increases lean body mass, decreases fatty tissue, helps fight the adverse effects of the heavy oxygen intake required by aerobic exercise, and even relieves the stress symptoms that many women suffer during menopause.

Well, there's a substance that just may offer all those benefits, and it's organic, too. Gama-oryzanol is a white powder extracted from rice bran oil. It was discovered more than 30 years ago by a Japanese researcher, but only recently has it come to the attention of a significant number of people who want to get more out of their workouts.

One of four variations known as *isomers* of a parent compound called *oryzanol*, GO (as gama-oryzanol is properly called) probably works on the hypothalamus in the brain, which has direct contact with the central nervous system. Through its control of the pituitary gland, the hypothalamus governs a number of your body's automatic functions, including temperature control, water balance, and hormonal regulation.

Those hormones include the sex hormones—testosterone in the male and estrogen in the female. It appears that GO may increase testosterone production, which would account for the increased lean body mass that researchers have observed in GO-fed lab animals. Fatty tissue, however, appears actually to decrease with the use of GO.

The final results aren't in yet, but it goes without saying that a safe and effective substance that stimulates growth would be welcomed enthusiastically by training athletes.

Another benefit of GO's hypothalamus connection may be its effect on female hormones. Women who have been administered GO in controlled experiments found that many of the distressful symptoms of menopause-related hormone imbalances were reduced.

GO has another and more immediate benefit to anybody who engages in regular and intense exercise. It acts as an antioxidant, meaning it helps to neutralize the chemical particles known as *free radicals* that are released in your body during heavy exercise. These free radicals have a detrimental effect on your system. They can be likened to incompletely burned chips or sparks of fuel (picture embers flying from smoldering fire wood) that shoot through your bloodstream.

Your body's production of energy for aerobic acitivity requires huge amounts of oxygen, which in turn creates these free radicals that tend to attach themselves to and damage cellular membranes.

Your body offsets this destructive activity by using antioxidant chemicals, which lock on to the free radicals and eliminate them. Vitamin E and selenium are two well-known antioxidants. GO is now another.

In fact, where GO is available as a supplement in health food stores, it is frequently found in a compound that combines 20 milligrams of GO with 100 international units of vitamin E. This one-to-five ratio produces the best results in free-radical protection.

How much GO should you take for free-radical protection and other benefits? Use the following as a guide.

Light-intensity training: 5 milligrams daily
Moderate-intensity training: 10 to 15 milligrams daily
High-intensity training: 20 to 30 milligrams daily, along with 100 to 150 international units of vitamin E and 50 micrograms of selenium.

23
ANTIOXIDANTS

Some interesting changes occur to your body as you increase the frequency or intensity of your exercise program. Most of these changes are beneficial, but some are stressful. Improper exercise, poor diet, and ignorance about how your body works can cause more damage than good.

Pay special attention—what you're about to read may be news to you, and it's not that easy to comprehend the first time around. The following discussion covers some advanced biochemistry concepts and explains some of the little-known but harmful effects of strenuous exercise. Once you grasp these basic concepts you'll know how to protect yourself while pushing your athletic performance limits.

Vigorous workouts can raise your muscles' need for oxygen by 20 times. This elevated muscle activity and raised oxygen demand can result in free-radical damage, hypoxia, and lactate accumulation. These three conditions are interrelated in a complex series of processes triggered by strenuous exercise.

Free-Radical Damage

Free radicals are highly unstable, reactive and dangerous chemical molecular fragments that damage proteins and other cells of your body upon contact. There is evidence that free radicals can cause genetic damage and even cancer. Exercise stimulates production of two main types of these chemicals: oxygen radicals and peroxide radicals.

Oxygen radicals are incompletely burned stages of oxygen, like sparks in a fireplace. Peroxide radicals are organic particles formed when damage occurs to the parts of cells made up of polyunsaturated fats. This damage can be caused by several factors, including contact with oxygen radicals, which triggers a chain reaction of destruction to fat cells.

Peroxide radicals disrupt your cell membranes as well as cell proteins that carry out metabolic functions. Also, peroxide radicals break down into other products that are worse than the free radicals themselves in terms of destructive potential.

Lactate Accumulation

Another harmful by-product of strenuous exercise is lactic acid buildup, brought about by the anaerobic breakdown of glycogen in the muscle fibers. This accumulation of lactate must be filtered by the liver in a process that requires increased oxygen. When your liver cannot clean up lactate fast enough, the lactate accumulates to the point where you feel fatigued and want to quit exercising.

Hypoxia

Your increased training efforts can also lead to hypoxia, or lack of oxygen, which affects your muscles, liver, and various other organs and tissues. If you keep on working out after your oxygen levels drop, your cells will respond by producing lactate because they are forced to break down glycogen for energy fuel. Your cells can no longer use oxygen to produce energy.

Overabundance of lactate damages proteins in the muscle cells by making the surrounding tissue very acidic. As your muscle cells deplete their glycogen stores, they resort to burning proteins for fuel, stressing your kidneys.

Hypoxia can cause your muscles and other cells to leak calcium, which interferes with your endurance. Hypoxia in the pituitary gland can cause amenorrhea (cessation of the menstrual cycle) in women who train hard. "Runner's anemia" or "sports anemia" (the breakdown of red blood cells) is caused by pituitary hypoxia.

This lack of oxygen produces free radicals and can cause your tissues to digest themselves from the inside. This damages the proteins and, combined with a return to normal oxygen levels after you've finished exercising, produces another kind of free radical called a *superoxide*. The superoxide attacks the cell membrane, thus generating peroxide free radicals and starting the chain reaction of cell destruction.

As we can see, lactate buildup and hypoxia cause not only direct damage to cells but also indirect destruction as they start the formation of free radicals.

It is in the mitochondria, the "powerhouses" of the cells, that most free radicals are formed when oxygen is used to burn glucose or other fuels. During this fuel-burning process, about 3 to 5 percent of incompletely burned oxygen escapes as oxygen free radicals. As these "sparks" land on the membranes of the mitochondria, they react with the polyunsaturated fats to create peroxide free radicals.

When you're not working out, these free radicals don't cause any problem because your body protects its cells with natural antioxidants. It's when you're exercising and using 5 to 20 times more oxygen than usual that free radicals break through the cell membranes of the mitochondria and wreak havoc. Free radicals damage other parts of your cells, including DNA, and invade the bloodstream. Peroxide levels in the plasma rise to twice the levels at rest, potentially creating other toxic and inflammatory substances.

What are the consequences? It's amazing that all this destruction of cells and bloodstream doesn't cause you more problems. The truth is, most of the effects of these reactions are noticed by beginners. Muscle pains, cramps, and other uncomfortable symptoms associated with "lactate poisoning" are the most common manifestations of these exercise-induced reactions. As your body gets used to the increased intensity or length of your exercise sessions, the noticeable effects are reduced.

Over the long term, this chain reaction of effects can lead to excessive weight loss, dehydration, muscle burnout, anemia, and negative nitrogen balance. Research so far is inconclusive on the possible link between exercise and DNA damage and cancer. It may be that people who exercise have a lower risk of DNA damage or cancer, because athletes tend to take good care of their health in general.

How to Protect Yourself

Fortunately, your body has natural defenses against damage from free radicals: antioxidants in the form of vitamins C and E and other biochemicals. Vitamin E wipes out peroxide free radicals in membranes, and vitamin C destroys oxygen radicals and other water-soluble free radicals.

Other antioxidants are vitamin A, uric acid, and enzymes such as glutathione peroxidase (which contains selenium) and superoxide dismutase (SOD).

There are steps you can take in your Ultimate Sports Nutrition diet and exercise programs to enhance your antioxidant defenses. The type and intensity of training you do determines what protection you need. Endurance exercise such as long-distance running and cycling produces moderate to high levels of free radicals in the mitochondria but doesn't seriously damage other parts of the cells and other tissues. However, sprint and strength types of exercise, such as weightlifting and tennis, can create more widespread damage.

Here are some tips to strengthen your defenses against free-radical damage:

- Ironic as it may seem, regular exercise is one of your best defenses against exercise-induced free-radical damage. People who are consistent in their workout programs have more resistance to lactate buildup and hypoxia and reduced damage from exercise-induced oxidation than people who don't engage in physical activity. This is why beginners seem to suffer more ill effects than highly conditioned athletes whose systems have adapted to the effects of exercise.
- If you're just starting your exercise program, take it easy in the beginning and gradually increase the intensity and length of your workouts. Exercise about 15 minutes a day until your body gets used to the new program. Oxidative damage is sure to occur if you exercise too intensely at first.
- Consume sufficient calories so that your body doesn't burn its own protein for fuel. Being underweight is a greater health risk than being overweight when you need lots of energy for exercise.
- Supplement your diet with 800 international units of vitamin E and up to 5,000 milligrams of vitamin C per day. Vitamin C needs to be accompanied by vitamin E, or else free radicals are generated—the opposite of the desired reaction.
- Include vitamin B_6 to reduce any effects of protein burning on the kidneys. Take some vitamin A too, but don't take megadoses of it or else hypoxialike side effects may occur.

110

• Selenium supplements build up the natural antioxidant glutathione peroxidase. For the time being, don't depend on orgotein,
the commercially available form of superoxide dismutase
(SOD), because research shows that SOD may not be effective
when taken orally.

You can buy commercial antioxidants in many health food stores.

111

PART FOUR
SPECIAL PROGRAMS
FOR ATHLETES

24
GAINING WEIGHT

As you leaf through back issues of bodybuilding magazines, you are bound to be struck by the awesome improvements in today's bodybuilding champions. "John Grimek couldn't win a local show if he were competing today," you say.

Shame on you! This is blasphemy! To disparage one of the greatest bodybuilders of all time is heresy! Yet it's true: bodybuilders today are more massive, more defined, more cut, more muscular, more everything.

For those of you who aren't bodybuilders but need to up your muscle mass for other sports, remember that today's athletes are bigger, stronger, and better trained than ever, as well.

Reasons abound: more sophisticated training methods, more genetic talent from a larger pool of athletes, financial support for training, a better understanding of diet and supplementing, and more drugs.

Don't get hung up on the last reason, though. Sure, drugs work to build muscular mass and strength, but they're certainly not the chief reason that today's superstars would beat the best of yesteryear.

No, I believe the answer lies in careful training methods coupled with nutritional supplementation and dieting. The science of creating muscle mass is light-years ahead of the pioneers' simple routines of lifting weights for three sets of 10 repetitions or alternating light and heavy workouts.

By studying the scientific principles of modern bodybuilding nutrition, you can understand why today's physique champions are superior to the stars of yesteryear. If you're a competitive body-builder or an athlete in any sport, you can apply these principles and techniques to your next competition training period.

114

Nutrition for Muscular Mass

Mass training is taking your body to its ultimate of adaptive stress in order to build usable muscular size. It means going beyond all bounds of intensity to coax every last muscle fiber to the limits of its potential in growth and development. It means moving heavier iron than you ever dreamed possible, often two or three times a day, every day, every week.

To undertake such a training regimen, my friend, you're gonna need help!

Calories and Discipline

Sitting on your derriere and stuffing yourself with 3,500 calories a day more than what your body needs will make you gain about one pound a day. Most of that will be fat due to your inactivity.

But to put on a pound of muscle, you must consume prodigious amounts of extra calories a day and *train like you've never trained before*. Then, if you've done everything right, you can expect to add a pound of muscle in a week or two. (See the table in this chapter for approximate time by body weight it takes to develop muscle mass.)

You must consume between 2,500 and 10,000 calories more than what your body ordinarily needs to add just one pound of muscle. No slack for us ironheads, friends. Just hard training, eating right, and self-discipline.

Self-discipline—the old-timers had it, probably as much as to-day's athletes. The old-timers sometimes refer derisively to today's athletes as "hothouse" athletes because the younger generation tends to take shortcuts for speedy growth of muscle. They are on an endless search for the magic potion, the secret formula for instant success. Drugs weren't as abundant in the old days, so athletes back then had to make huge sacrifices in time and effort to achieve greatness.

In many cases I agree with the old-timers, for there are indeed many shortcut athletes out there. But the old-timers fail to acknowledge the impressive strides today's champions have made. To be a champion today takes just as much sacrifice, dedication, discipline, and desire as before—even more, because the competition today is tougher.

Discipline means doing what is necessary to win: practicing scientific training techniques and following a controlled supplementation and diet program.

The maxim "You are what you eat" applies to athletes more so than to any other group. Each milligram of muscle tissue and each drop of blood in your body is formed from the nutrients you ingest in the food you eat every day. Unless you eat the types and quantities of foods that your body needs to increase muscle mass and strength, you won't make big gains. It's that simple.

The most important mass- and power-building nutrient is protein, which makes up the building blocks of muscle tissue. You must eat plenty of protein, and it must be of high biological quality. And, of course, you must observe healthful dietary practices to keep your body tuned up and free from nutritional deficiencies.

To review some nutritional basics explained in other chapters, the protein in human muscle tissue contains 22 amino acids, of which 12 are manufactured within the body. The other 10 "essential" amino acids must be contained in the foods that you eat each day. Only proteins from animal sources—meat, fish, chicken, eggs, and milk products—contain high levels of all essential amino acids. Vegetable-source proteins are either low or entirely lacking in one or more essential aminos. Therefore, your mass- and power-building diet should be high in animal-source proteins and supplemented with amino acids in order to improve the average protein efficiency ratio.

Lowfat or nonfat milk is a traditional favorite food among hard-training athletes. Many people cannot tolerate milk products due to deficiency of lactase, the enzyme that helps to digest lactose, or milk sugar. A common symptom of lactose intolerance or allergy is bloating. If you have this problem, try a special type of milk in which the lactose is predigested or add lactase pills or powder to your milk. These products are sold in health food stores.

The more protein your body is able to digest and assimilate, the larger and stronger your muscles can become in the days between heavy workouts. But your stomach can digest only about 25 to 30 grams of protein at each feeding. This means you can digest only 75 to 90 grams of protein per day if you eat three meals a day.

The Recommended Number of Weeks Required to Gain Muscle Weight					
Increase Desired (in pounds)	Present Lean Body Weight (in pounds)	Number of Weeks	Increase Desired (in pounds)	Present Lean Body Weight (in pounds)	Number of Weeks
5	100	10	20	100	40
	120	9.5		120	38
	140	9		140	36
	160	8.5		160	34
	180	8		180	32
	200	7.5		200	30
	220	7		220	28
	240	6.5		240	26
	260	6		260	24
	280	5.5		280	22
	300	5		300	20
10	100	20	25	100	50
	120	19		120	47.5
	140	18		140	45
	160	17		160	42.5
	180	16		180	40
	200	15		200	37.5
	220	14		220	35
	240	13		240	32.5
	260	12		260	30
	280	11		280	27.5
	300	10		300	25
15	100	30	30	100	60
	120	28.5		120	57
	140	27		140	54
	160	25.5		160	51
	180	24		180	48
	200	22.5		200	45
	220	21		220	42
	240	19.5		240	39
	260	18		260	36
	280	16.5		280	33
	300	15		300	30

Eating More Meals per Day

By eating five or six smaller meals per day, you can increase the amount of protein available for assimilation into muscle tissue. Each meal should include about 25 to 30 grams of animal-source protein. Eating more protein than that may result in its being stored as fat. (See Part V for suggested mass-building meals and snacks.)

Shakes

A fast and convenient way to up your protein intake and assimilation is to drink a high-protein shake two or three times a day. Instructions on how to make these delicious, low-calorie blender drinks are found in Part V.

Weight-Gain Tips

1. Eat dried fruits for an energy boost (but not just before a workout). Unsalted nuts and seeds are good, concentrated foods, but eat them in moderation because of their high fat content.
2. Load up on complex carbohydrates (rice, corn, pasta, potatoes, whole grain breads and cereals, beans, peas). Don't load these powerhouse foods with fatty spreads or sweet toppings, because fat slows digestion.
3. For desserts and snacks, eat breads made with fruits, whole grain flours, and natural sweeteners instead of oily pastries or frosted cakes. Carrot cake, banana bread, and oatmeal cookies are good choices—they contain beneficial fiber.
4. Fruit juice quenches thirst and supplies calories and potassium, a mineral vital to muscular action but lost during high-intensity workouts.
5. Add a bedtime snack for extra weight gain. If low in sugar, it won't keep you awake.
6. If you begin your day with an early-morning workout, drink a glass of juice before training. Afterward, have a good breakfast (pancakes with molasses or fresh fruit syrup, eggs with whole grain bread, yogurt with fruit and nuts). The juice supplies energy for your workout; a hearty breakfast replenishes calories burned during your workout.
7. See the "Nutrition For Muscular Definition" chapter for details on muscle mass improvement.

25
LOSING WEIGHT

There are two ways to lose weight: dehydrating to "make weight" for an athletic contest (discussed in Chapter 29) and losing fat to achieve your peak condition in health and appearance. This chapter deals with the latter way of losing weight.

There is no shortage of fad diet books to help you (and your wallet) weigh less. But some of the most popular diet methods—the Beverly Hills, Cambridge, Atkins, and Stillman diets—could be dangerous to your health if followed for an extended period of time.

The only safe way to lose weight and keep it off is to exercise properly and follow a balanced diet. The diet must contain sufficient calories, fiber, vitamins, and minerals to power you through your activities and keep you feeling good. Your food intake can be adjusted according to the amount of calories you burn during exercise.

Exercise Is the Key

The problem with losing weight is that there are so many misconceptions about how to do it. Recent research overturns our most popular and persistent myths regarding diet, exercise, and weight loss. One misconception is that exercise increases hunger. This is not true: studies show that exercise, if anything, initially *decreases* appetite.

Vigorous exercise continues to have an effect on your body for a time following the workout—it actually *suppresses* appetite for up to several hours afterward. Furthermore, exercise acts on another level to assist in weight loss: it releases tensions and anxieties, common triggers for overeating.

"Dieting"—by which we often mean restricting food intake to lose weight—carries a negative connotation because it is associated with depriving yourself of something you like. While not ignoring the nutritional aspect of losing weight, let's concentrate our discussion here on exercise. You probably will get better results in losing weight if you increase your exercise program, for exercise is active and positive. Exercising means spending time *doing something*, filling up time with activity, not restraining yourself from activity, as "dieting" suggests.

It's not just for psychological reasons that I recommend exercising for losing weight. Exercising burns calories; the more you exercise, the more calories you burn and the more pounds you lose. Lack of exercise is linked directly to obesity. Research shows that the beginning of obesity with humans can be traced to a sudden decrease in their activity levels. With animals it is the same story: to fatten up hogs and cattle for market, ranchers pen up the animals to restrict their movements while feeding them the same or even lesser amounts of food.

Another myth about losing weight is that exercise doesn't use enough calories to burn off very much fat. This may seem to be true, if you look at it on a superficial level. After all, according to mathematical calculations, you must walk 30 miles or play volleyball for 11 hours to burn just one pound of fat, It follows that walking or playing volleyball for one hour results in an insignificant amount of weight loss.

Well, not exactly. A little bit of weight loss per day, multiplied by many days, equals a significant number of pounds lost. We're talking here about training yourself in healthful, effective eating and exercise patterns to last your whole lifetime, not crashing off a few pounds of water bloat.

The long-term effect of regular, vigorous physical exercise is dramatic: it raises your basal metabolism rate, or the rate at which your body burns calories at rest. Thus, after you finish working out, your body is burning up to 15 percent more calories per hour for a period of several hours. Add this to the calories burned during exercise, and you've got some impressive statistics.

And don't forget about those peaks in exercise when you're

burning up to 1,500 calories per hour. These peaks aren't recorded on the standard calorie expenditure charts. Take a cross-country skier, for example, who can expend 4,000 to 5,000 calories in a three-hour workout. This is more calories than some people eat in three days! So you see, certain activities can result in a huge calorie deficit.

Set Point Theory

There is another important factor in losing weight: your "set point." "Set point" is that particular weight to which your body returns naturally when you aren't trying to restrict calories. Your body has its own level of fat that it wants to store, regardless of slight variations in day-to-day caloric intake and expenditure. You can manipulate your set point to a lower level by upping your aerobic exercise on a regular basis. Aerobic exercise makes your body hang on to less fat, and you will achieve this fat loss without stress to your psyche or body.

The opposite is also true: eating fats and sweets raises your set point, or the amount of fat your body strives to store.

Weight Loss Principles

In trying to lose weight, it helps to understand the scientific principles involved in the process. You already know that to lose one pound of fat (3,500 calories), your food intake must be 3,500 calories less than your usual calorie expenditure.

This may seem to suggest a brutally slow process, but there are other factors in the picture.

Water and Fat Loss

For the first two weeks of a reduced-calorie diet, up to 70 percent of the initial weight loss is in the form of water. As your body burns its most accessible fuel—the glycogen stored in muscles—it releases three or four grams of water for each gram of glycogen. For the first two weeks of a low-calorie diet, you may lose three or more pounds per week.

This is a dramatic amount of weight loss, and it should encourage you to stick with your diet.

It isn't until about two weeks into your reduced-calorie diet that your body starts burning fat. Because fat contains many more calories per pound than glycogen, it takes longer to lose fat. This is the toughest part of your weight-loss diet because, after two weeks, there is less water loss. At this two- or three-week point, it takes extra resolve to stick to your diet. The pounds come off more slowly—only one or two pounds per week—and it's easy to get discouraged.

But don't dive in to the temptation to starve yourself in an attempt to lose pounds faster—an ultra-low-calorie diet lacks food variety, vitamins, and minerals your body needs to perform at its maximum level.

After the first two or three weeks of your diet, it's critical that you exercise. This is because your body will start to convert protein from lean tissue into energy—actually burning up muscles for energy. Unless you are exercising, your muscle mass will diminish on a reduced-calorie diet. Exercise keeps your muscles toned and intact in size.

Be sure to exercise if you go off your diet for a few days so that you'll continue to burn calories and not gain weight. If you do gain, the pounds will be fat, not muscle. Stay active!

Metabolism Adaptations

The body has an interesting survival mechanism that can backfire on your weight-loss goals. If you try to lose weight by severely restricting your caloric intake instead of adopting a moderate diet, your body will perceive this as a threat to its survival and respond by slowing its metabolism to save energy.

So you can eat almost nothing and still not lose weight, because your body will drastically slow down its metabolic rate. A low-calorie diet also makes your body more efficient at storing fat, which is counter to your goals.

So it all comes back to exercise as the key to losing weight. Working out burns calories, reduces your set point, and adds fun to your fitness program. It most certainly is necessary in achieving peak athletic performance.

No Weight Loss

If you don't start losing weight after adopting an exercise program, don't worry. The exercise might be toning your muscles or building muscle mass, which could result in more muscular size while you weigh the same—or even more. Just stay with your diet and exercise program. After the muscle growth stabilizes, you'll eventually start losing fat.

So far nobody has discovered a better way to lose weight than to follow a reduced-calorie diet comprised of at least three to four meals per day and an increased exercise program. No matter how you go about it, starving yourself just doesn't work.

Aerobic Exercise

Exercises that burn fat the fastest are the aerobic ones: running, cycling, skating, cross-country skiing, rowing, swimming. Don't forget other sports that demand bursts of anaerobic energy, such as tennis, racquetball, soccer, basketball, and volleyball.

Weight training can be an aerobic activity, if performed without resting between sets. Aerobic weight training, also called *circuit training*, usually is done with one set per exercise, quickly going from one station or exercise to the next, without the customary 30- to 90-second rest between sets. Exercising like this keeps the heart rate within target range and creates the "training effect" of improved cardiovascular efficiency.

An added benefit of lifting weights to lose body fat is that weight training builds muscles—and larger muscles burn more calories than smaller ones. (Fat seems not to burn any calories at all—it just sits in lumps on the body.)

Weight training develops the muscles to their normal size. In most sports, developed muscles are advantageous, for a high strength-to-weight ratio means lower body fat and improved muscle mass and strength. These factors result in improved sports performance.

Carbohydrates and Glycemic Index

As you read in the chapter on carbohydrates (also see Chapter 30, on carbohydrate loading), carbohydrates provide fuel for energy faster and more efficiently than fats or proteins. This is due to their relative Glycemic Index, or rate at which blood sugar rises and drops after eating the food. Use the accompanying table to select carbohydrate foods with a *low* Glycemic Index—that is, 50 and below. These foods convert to blood sugar at a slower and more even rate, providing you with a steady supply of fuel for exercise.

Foods with a high Glycemic Index (over 50) are mostly simple carbohydrates that give you a sudden burst of energy, only to cause an abrupt drop in blood sugar that leaves you tired, light-headed, and hungry. The way to lose weight is to make wise eating choices that don't leave you with hunger pangs. Before workouts or competition, avoid foods with a Glycemic Index of more than 50.

Thermogenesis

One way to burn calories is to stimulate your body's core temperature to rise, a condition called *thermogenesis*. This can be done by keeping cool, which provokes a shivering response, your body's signal to burn calories to create body heat. Swimming in cold water is thermogenic, as is staying in a chilly, air-conditioned room.

Weight-Loss Regimen

To assist you in your weight-loss goals, I have prepared a simple list of diet tips inspired by the bestselling book *The Life Extension Weight Loss Program*, by Durk Pearson and Sandy Shaw.

1. Take growth hormone releasers—ornithine, arginine, niacin, methionine, tryptophan—*before training and before bed.*
2. Eat carbohydrates with low Glycemic Index (under 50).
3. Substitute fructose for sucrose (table sugar).
4. Take chromium supplements for blood sugar and insulin regulation.
5. Curb appetite immediately before meals with caffeine, high-protein powder, and L-phenylalanine in the morning with vitamins C and B_6.
6. Eat high-fiber foods as often as possible.
7. Take L-carnitine supplements regularly.
8. Drink Ma Huang tea with fructose once a day for thermogenesis.
9. Stay cool—don't wear bundles of clothing. Lower temperatures are thermogenic.
10. Keep accurate records (at least weekly) of all body measurements.
11. Train with weights very hard for a half hour or more every day. Alternate your forms of exercise: for example, cycle one day, weight train the next, take an aerobic class the third, etc.

26
MAKING WEIGHT FOR COMPETITION

If you compete in bodybuilding, powerlifting, wrestling, and boxing, you're familiar with the weigh-in prior to the contest to ensure that you are pitted fairly against opponents of your weight class. Obviously, you have an advantage if you keep your body weight at the high end of a weight class rather than at the bottom of the next higher weight class. You want to be as heavy as possible in your weight class because contest results show irrefutably that athletes perform better this way.

Maintaining that fine line between "making weight" and exceeding can be a hassle for many of us! Most of the time, making weight means we have to drop a few pounds to qualify for our weight class. Dropping a few pounds is done only for major events, for three or four meets that really matter during a competitive season. Don't bother losing weight for minor meets or training events or if doing so won't make any difference in how you place. In those cases, stay at your normal body weight.

Dropping weight is tricky business. The trick is to shed the pounds without shedding even one smidgen of performance in the contest. By following the guidelines explained in this chapter, you'll be able to lose those pounds safely while maintaining your performance capabilities.

Pounds Lost	Beginning Body Weight (before weight loss)									
	120	140	160	180	200	220	240	260	280	300
1	0	0	0	0	0	0	0	0	0	0
2	0	0	0	0	0	0	0	0	0	0
3	0	0	0	0	0	0	0	0	0	0
4	1	0	0	0	0	0	0	0	0	0
5	2.5	1	0	0	0	0	0	0	0	0
6	4	2.5	1	0	0	0	0	0	0	0
7	5.5	4	2.5	1	0	0	0	0	0	0
8	7	5.5	4	2.5	1	0	0	0	0	0
9	8.5	7	5.5	4	2.5	1	0	0	0	0
10	10	8.5	7	5.5	4	2.5	1	0	0	0
11	11.5	10	8.5	7	5.5	4	2.5	1	0	0
12	13	11.5	10	8.5	7	5.5	4	2.5	1	0
13	14.5	13	11.5	10	8.5	7	5.5	4	2.5	1
14	17	14.5	13	11.5	10	8.5	7	5.5	4	2.5
15	18.5	17	14.5	13	11.5	10	8.5	7	5.5	4
16	20	18.5	16	14.5	13	11.5	10	8.5	7	5.5
17	21.5	20	18.5	16	14.5	13	11.5	10	8.5	7
18	23	21.5	20	18.5	16	14.5	13	11.5	10	8.5
19	24.5	23	21.5	20	18.5	16	14.5	13	11.5	10
20	26	24.5	23	21.5	20	18.5	16	14.5	13	11.5
	Strength Lost in Pounds from Lift									

Stay Within Limits

During the off-season, keep your training weight within 3.5 percent of the class limit. This allows you to drop the few pounds necessary to make weight without suffering any strength loss whatsoever. For every pound lost above this allowable limit, you can expect to lose strength.

For example, a powerlifter will lose about 1.5 pounds from each lift for each pound of body weight shed beyond the 3.5 percent limit. In the table opposite, check out how much weaker you will be according to how many pounds you drop before a contest.

127

Lose Water, Not Muscle Mass

The pounds you shed to make weight should be from water. The simplest way to do this is to sweat off the extra pounds in a sauna or steam room. Bear in mind that sweat sessions can be psychologically and physically draining, so do a few sessions way in advance of the contest to get accustomed to the effects.

The absolute worst way to make weight is to crash-diet down. If you're heavier than the 3.5 percent limit in your desired weight class, you should have been dieting for weeks and months prior to the weigh-in. Making weight means dropping only a few pounds at the last minute, not making major changes.

Dieting down causes even greater decrements in performance than those predicted in the table above. Fasting, for example, will result in weight loss—but it will be 65 percent from muscle and 35 percent from fat and water in the first 10 days of dieting. Losing that much muscle inevitably causes devastating declines in your strength—and you simply won't perform at your best level during the contest. Summon up all the discipline you can muster to keep your body weight within the prescribed limits. If you can't use good, old-fashioned discipline to achieve your athletic goals, you're in the wrong field, buddy. Take up stamp collecting.

Diuretics

Diuretics used by athletes wishing to drop a few pounds of water weight are commonly prescription medications that stimulate urination. A common brand used by athletes is Lasix. If you are within the 3.5 percent limit and sweating doesn't get rid of enough water weight, try taking diuretics according to the following instructions, but *only* in consultation with your physician:

1. Do not skip meals. The weight will come off, so don't panic by fasting. Just eat less at each meal.
2. If you need to lose more than 3.5 percent of body weight, do it during the last two or three days before the contest. This less-than-strenuous dieting plan is not psychologically traumatic and will allow you to lose only a minimal degree of strength.
3. If you take diuretics, potassium supplements, or any other medications, always follow the instructions and note the precautions, indications, and contraindications. Listen to your doctor.
4. Following weigh-in, replace fluids according to the instructions outlined below.

Electrolyte Replacement

Dropping water weight increases the risk of depleting your body of its required mineral stores, including potassium. Thanks to all the research that's been done over the past few years, you can steer yourself in the right direction to avoid dehydration and mineral loss during your attempts to make weight.

Sweating off excess water is the preferred mode of making weight, but you need to know what else you're losing along with the water. Take a look at the accompanying table.

Electrolytes (mEq/liter)

	Sodium	Chloride	Potassium	Magnesium	**TOTAL**
Plasma	140	100	4	1.5	145.5
Sweat	40–60	30–50	4–5	1.5–5	75.5–120

Profuse sweating affects the concentration of electrolytes in your blood, for sweat is actually a filtrate of blood plasma. Losing electrolytes during perspiration causes you to lose more water than electrolytes from the plasma, leaving the plasma more concentrated. After sweating, your need for water is greater than your need for electrolytes. Drink plenty of water, and drink it cold, because cold water is assimilated into the bloodstream faster than warm or tepid water.

Recent research has found that sports drinks containing carbohydrates (glucose) and sodium, such as Gatorade Thirst Quencher, can be effective fluid replacement beverages, because they are quickly absorbed in the small intestine.

Whatever electrolyte replacement therapy you choose, do it before you start sweating. Or, if you must sweat off some pounds to make weight at the contest site, drink a dilute form (half water) of the beverage. Consume the drink at 10- to 15-minute intervals, in quantities not exceeding 400 milliliters (10 ounces). Stop drinking when you have replaced lost fluids and eat a good meal after the contest to replace lost electrolytes.

129

How To Prevent Cramps

Consuming fluids before exercising has a drawback—it may cause cramps. Cramps are more likely to occur if your sports drink is full of sugar, too concentrated, tepid or warm and if you consume too much. Cramps may plague you if you don't replace electrolytes prior to competition. Be careful if you use diuretics, because they cause loss of electrolytes, which increases your chances of cramping.

Mauro DiPasquale, M.D., a powerlifter from Canada, has figured out a formula for the relationship among the various mineral ions in the body. The formula shows how an excess or a deficiency of minerals can lead to cramping:

$$\text{Tendency to cramp} = \frac{(K)\ (HCO)\ (HPO)}{(NA)\ (CA)\ (MG)\ (H)}$$

He has found that your muscles will tend to cramp if you lack sufficient calcium, magnesium, or sodium or if the plasma acidity is decreased, which is what happens with hyperventilation. Cramps also may be caused by an excess of certain minerals—potassium, phosphate, or sodium bicarbonate, which some nervous athletes take to reduce stomach acidity.

"The practical application of this interrelationship of minerals is wide," says DiPasquale. "For example, to reduce your tendency to cramp, you could increase calcium for several days prior to a contest. Another technique would be to try *not* to hyperventilate at contests. Also, don't use antacids, especially sodium bicarbonate, prior to a meet, because all antacids decrease plasma acidity."

Use of diuretics increases the risk of body potassium losses. You can prevent this by taking potassium supplements in the correct amounts—too much causes an imbalance of electrolyte concentrations in the blood, just as too little does. Diuretics are potentially dangerous substances; use them only under medical supervision.

"If you use diuretics to make weight, you face a double problem," says DiPasquale. "Most diuretics decrease the sodium content of the body. This, by itself, predisposes one to muscle cramps, because diuretics also decrease body potassium—which can lead to muscle weakness. So if you use diuretics, you should increase both your salt and potassium only moderately."

130

If cramping occurs during a contest, DiPasquale recommends a slightly acidic prepared solution containing calcium, magnesium, and sodium. "If this doesn't work," he says, "then you may be forced to use muscle relaxants prescribed by your physician. Regardless of which ones you choose, they'll all stun you to some extent and affect your athletic performance."

27
NUTRITION FOR MUSCULAR DEFINITION

Competitive bodybuilders are judged not only on muscular size but also on muscular definition, separation, and striation. You must look lean, cut, and ripped, with deep lines etched between muscles.

Most bodybuilders attempt to develop this cut-to-ribbons definition by rigidly restricting food and water intake the last week before a contest. Contrary to popular belief, it is counterproductive and potentially dangerous to severely reduce food and water intake. Achieving the finest possible degreee of muscle definition is the *easiest and most predictable part of creating a winning physique—especially in the last week before a competition.*

Approaching the Last Week

No matter how you alter your diet and exercise programs during the last week before a contest, you cannot be at your best unless you have trained and dieted properly beforehand. All you accomplish during the last week is to carb up, which allows you to show off your physique to its best advantage.

Your dieting should not be so severe that you lose muscle mass along with body fat; your metabolism slows down and thus becomes less efficient at burning body fat, or you lack the energy to train intensely.

It's inadvisable to diet for weight loss right up to the day of the contest. *Reach your contest weight or below at least a week before show time.* Rather than dieting away body fat the last week, simply start your diet program a week earlier. During the last week, follow the program outlined below, and you will maintain your body weight or even gain a couple of pounds.

Water Control

132

No matter what you've heard, the best way for you, whether you're male or female, to get into top contest shape is to *keep as much fat and water in the body as possible—as long as you still look ripped.*

Dieting away excessive amounts of body fat is a mistake because the bodybuilding physique, which carries an unusual amount of muscle, also contains larger-than-normal amounts of intramuscular fat. This internal fat contributes to both muscle size and muscle shape, and when you diet it away, you make yourself appear smaller and softer.

You're mistaken if you believe that you look more ripped and defined when you dehydrate your body. Certainly, you don't want a lot of subcutaneous water blurring the sharpness of your definition. But muscle is composed of more than 75 percent water, and each gram of glycogen your body stores as energy for muscular contraction binds with 2.7 grams of water. So the more water you have in your body, the bigger and harder you will look, *provided you can force that water into the muscles instead of letting it remain subcutaneous.*

There are two ways to push water into the muscle cells: altering the electrolyte balance across the cell membrane, inducing the water to go from extracellular to intracellular; and carbing up effectively, causing the body to absorb large amounts of glycogen along with three times as much water.

Sodium Loading

The water balance across the muscle cell membrane is regulated by the balance between potassium inside the cell and sodium outside. When there is an excess of potassium, water is drawn into the muscle cell. With an excess of sodium, water is drawn out of the cell.

You can force additional water into the muscle cell by changing its potassium/sodium balance. This is achieved by reducing sodium intake and taking potassium supplements.

Your body strives to maintain its potassium/sodium balance. When you restrict your sodium intake, the body begins to excrete potassium to restore the equality between the levels of the two minerals. Therefore, you should *restrict your sodium for about three days prior to a contest.* The problem is that staying on a low-sodium diet for several weeks will result in a lowering of your potassium levels, which inhibits that cut and ripped look for a contest.

The answer is to eat moderately high levels of sodium for a week or so prior to starting your low-sodium program. When you finally do reduce your sodium levels, you will have naturally high levels of potassium. This exaggerates the potassium/sodium imbalance and accelerates the transport of water into the muscle cells.

This sodium loading does not need to be excessive, and it should not be maintained for a long time because high sodium levels are associated with diseases such as hypertension. The sodium loading method is merely a short-term technique of temporarily causing the body to respond one way so that you can stimulate a more extreme reaction in the opposite direction.

Potassium Supplements

To move water out of the space between cells and into the cells, three days before a bodybuilding contest, add potassium supplements to your low-sodium diet. Exactly how much potassium to take is an individual matter. A 200-pound bodybuilder should take about 100 milligrams five times a day, for a total of 500 milligrams.

Never take potassium on an empty stomach, or you'll experience unpleasant side effects, such as nausea or upset stomach.

Carbing Up

Muscle size is determined only partially by hypertrophy, or growth, of muscle fibers. Another factor that adds to muscle size is blood supply to the muscles, delivered by the additional capillaries created by hard training. Also, muscle size is determined by the amount of glycogen the muscles are able to store.

Hard training and dieting for a contest leave your body glycogen-depleted. Because the body is programmed to overcompensate for most depletion conditions, it will be predisposed to store larger-than-normal amounts of glycogen. You can manipulate your diet to exaggerate this overcompensation even further.

133

This is done by restricting your carbohydrate intake for a period of about one week, or until your body goes into ketosis (a state of carbohydrate deprivation that indicates presence of ketones). In ketosis, your body will suck up carbohydrates like a vacuum. Normally, the body stores about 2 to 3 grams of glycogen for every 100 grams of muscle weight. But when you induce a state of carbohydrate deprivation, it can store 4 to 5 grams of glycogen per 100 grams of muscle weight. Then, about three days before the contest, you load up on high-carbohydrate foods.

This method of carbohydrate loading results in bigger, more shapely muscles. It stimulates huge amounts of water to combine with the glycogen, pumping up your muscles and pulling large amounts of water out from under the skin.

Don't make the mistake of most bodybuilders: insufficient carbing up. A 150-pound bodybuilder theoretically can store about 9,000 calories of carbohydrates, and a bigger person even more. While it is inadvisable to carb up to this degree (too much muscle glycogen tends to obscure muscle separation), you must take in more than a few hundred grams of carbs over a several-day period.

Because of physical differences such as muscular mass, overall body size, and rate of metabolism, it is difficult to say exactly how many carbs you need. Another variable is the degree of deprivation when you start this process. Here's a rule of thumb: a relatively small male bodybuilder should consume about 3,000 to 5,000 calories of carbohydrates per day prior to a contest.

Since the body cannot absorb excessive amounts of carbohydrates all at one time, the carbs should be eaten at a rate of about 100 calories per hour. One gram of carbohydrates yields about 4½ calories, so this means eating a minimum of about 25 grams of carbs per hour per day—the equivalent of a baked potato or two small oranges.

The body requires 72 hours or more to carbohydrate load fully. So start your carbing up process no later than the Wednesday evening before a Saturday contest. Stay on the high-carbohydrate diet for about three days. Women seem to carb up faster than men, perhaps because their larger percentage of body fat retains more water or because there is less muscle mass to absorb the grams of glycogen.

To ingest 4,000 total calories of carbs (1000 grams) in three days, you must take in 1,330 calories or 330 grams per day. This breaks down to our formula of 100 calories (25 grams) per hour over a 16-hour period, which, as explained above, is a manageable amount. Bigger bodybuilders can increase their total carbohydrate consumption by taking in a higher hourly amount. But don't stuff yourself full at one sitting!

Eat only high-quality, complex carbs—those rich in vitamins, minerals, and fiber and low in fat and sugar: fruits, baked potatoes, rice, whole grains, raw green vegetables. Lay off high-sodium foods. Avoid processed sugar because it stimulates production of insulin, which results in edema, or subcutaneous water retention.

135

Training

Bodybuilding training burns up large amounts of muscle glycogen. Therefore, during the carbohydrate-depletion phase, it makes sense to train hard. But during the carbing-up period, conserve the muscle glycogen you've accumulated. If you start carbing up Wednesday for a Saturday contest, do high-repetition training Sunday through Wednesday, then intense posing Thursday through Saturday.

Posing is the best type of exercise prior to a contest, because flexing your muscles won't burn up a lot of glycogen but does make the muscles harder and more defined. Also, it helps you build the endurance you will need for long periods of posing on stage.

During the carbing-up phase, aerobic exercise should be kept to no more than 45 minutes per day in order to maximize muscle mass. More aerobics than this tends to reduce muscle size. (The carbohydrate-depletion phase is when aerobics is beneficial to the competitive bodybuilder.) Light aerobic activity prior to the show is all right; it works to stimulate your basal metabolism without burning up large amounts of your muscle glycogen.

Steroids and Other Drugs

A side effect of anabolic steroids, especially those with high androgenic indices, is water retention. Users of steriods and certain other medications, such as cortisone, experience bloating and have trouble attaining that super-ripped shape.

Prevent water retention by avoiding these drugs. The carbohydrate-depletion process results in a temporary state of dehydration, which should circumvent edema. If, however, you find yourself retaining excessive subcutaneous water in the three days prior to a show, follow the carbing-up process as described above—with one change. Cut down drastically on the amount of water you drink. This will cause the body to draw the subcutaneous water into the muscle cells. Once your muscles start appearing defined, increase your water intake to allow the carbing-up/water-binding process to proceed.

Bodybuilding Competition: The Final-Week Training Schedule

Sunday Through Wednesday Evening

High-repetition weight training
Moderate aerobics
Medium to high sodium
Low carbohydrates

Wednesday Evening Through Saturday

Little or no weight training
Intense posing
Low or no aerobics
Carbing up (100 calories per hour)
Low sodium
Plenty of distilled water
Potassium supplements

28
EATING FOR ENDURANCE

If you're an endurance athlete, your nutritional needs are greater than those of strength athletes. Your food intake is called upon several times a day to rebuild and repair body tissues that get broken down by exercise at a rate 5 to 10 times your normal resting rate.

Compared to recreational and strength athletes, you must be the most systematic and conscientious in maintaining a sound nutritional program. The typically haphazard American diet simply won't cut it in your strenuous training program. You need to monitor your diet to make sure you're getting the right foods in the right amounts for the functions of fueling, tissue repair, and regulation of body processes.

Fuel Foods

Although your body can use proteins, fats, or carbohydrates for energy, some foods make better fuel for endurance exercise than other foods. By far the best source of energy fuel is complex carbohydrates, from which your glycogen stores in the muscles are derived, as is the sugar circulating in the blood (blood glucose). As you use up your blood glucose, your liver provides fuel by breaking down and releasing into the blood some of its stored glycogen.

Blood-borne fats provide the next most accessible energy fuel. Some fat is stored in the muscles, but most fat is stored in the fat cells in the form of triglycerides. After your muscle glycogen stores are depleted, these triglycerides are broken down into free fatty acids (FFAs) and released into the blood, where they are absorbed into the muscles and burned for energy.

Protein is last on the list of preferred energy sources, for it is not stored for fuel like carbohydrates and fats. To be used as fuel for exercise, the body's muscle protein first must be broken down into amino acids and transported to the liver. There the amino acids are converted to glucose, which is released into the blood and used by the cells as fuel.

What type of fuel do you burn during exercise? The answer depends upon several factors, mainly the duration and intensity of the activity. What's important to know is that your performance capabilities may be limited by the sizes of your various fuel stores.

Your muscles and liver have limited capacities for storing glycogen. The limit seems to be 1½ to 2 hours of endurance exercise, after which the glycogen stores are depleted and your blood sugar level plummets. The sudden drop in energy feels like "hitting the wall" or "bonking," terms used by marathoners and distance cyclists to describe the abrupt and devastating letdown in energy.

So it's easy to use up significant amounts of your muscle and liver glycogen in two hours or less. But it's impossible to deplete your fat stores. Marathoner Alberto Salazar, for example, has a body fat level of 8 or 9 percent, or about 12 to 13½ pounds of his 150-pound body weight. Let's say 5 pounds of this is essential body weight. This gives him 7 to 8½ pounds of stored fat to use during his race. Since 1 pound of fat provides about 3,500 calories, his fat theoretically provides him with enough energy to run almost 35 miles—much more than a marathon distance!

The problem is that fat cannot be used as a fuel unless some carbohydrates are present in the muscle cells and liver. So a marathoner cannot run for miles on his supply of fat after his glycogen stores have been depleted. As an endurance athlete, you must figure out a nutritional plan that allows you to use your glycogen sparingly so that your fat stores serve as the main fuel source.

Protein is not intended to serve as a primary fuel source. Yet, if your blood glucose is depleted during the latter portions of a long race, your body will break down muscle protein to maintain blood glucose levels. Protein is an extremely inefficient and expensive fuel source.

The best nutritional plan for burning fuel for endurance activity is to maximize glycogen storage, use fats instead of glycogen, and minimize use of protein. Here's how you can achieve this strategy:

1. *Train for endurance on a regular basis.* The highly conditioned athlete can store about twice the amount of muscle glycogen and has 1½ times more intramuscular fat than the average sedentary person. Training also increases the size and number of mitochondria (the structures in cells where fats and carbohydrates are burned) as well as the enzymes (chemicals) needed for burning fats.

2. *Eat frequent and regularly spaced meals that emphasize complex carbohydrates (50 to 70 percent) and are low in fats (30 percent or less).* To keep body weight low, eat several small meals rather than one or two large ones. Eating carbohydrates frequently helps keep your blood glucose levels high and stimulates insulin release, which is needed for glycogen storage.

   Eat two to three hours after exercising, when your hormonal environment assists glycogen storage. Exercise releases hormones that help break down chemicals in your body.

   Don't be erratic in your carbohydrate consumption. Your body needs carbs on a regular daily basis during hard training. If your carbohydrate consumption dips to 40 percent or below, your muscle glycogen stores will gradually drop, and training will be a drag. Make sure your carbohydrates are of the complex type, for research suggests that they maximize glycogen storage better than simple sugars do.

3. *Avoid fat loading.* Discovering that the metabolism of fat contributes most of the energy for endurance activities, some researchers have experimented with placing elite athletes on high-fat diets. The results suggest that this is a dangerous and even life-threatening practice—although it will increase endurance. The five elite cyclists were fed a 4,000-calorie diet consisting of less than 5 percent carbohydrates for four weeks. The cyclists reported they could pedal longer before exhaustion set in.

   But the researchers found that the cyclists' cholesterol levels soared 15 to 20 percent, which increases the risk of heart problems. Also, the increased urine production caused by high-fat diets is associated with substantial losses of potassium, potentially leading to cardiac arrhythmias. Therefore, fat loading is not recommended as a sound nutritional practice for endurance athletes—or anyone else.

4. *Restrict carbohydrate consumption, including sugared beverages, 1½ to 2 hours before endurance activities.* Carbohydrate digestion suppresses mobilization and use of free fatty acids. This means your muscle glycogen stores will be used as fuel for the first part of the exercise session—and you'll get tired faster. Remember, your goals are to spare muscle glycogen stores and maximize use of fats as fuel.

5. *Eat carbohydrates during endurance exercise.* Once exercise begins, release of insulin is suppressed. Eating carbohydrates during exercise spares the use of glycogen in the liver and muscles and allows fat to be used as fuel.

   Drinking sugared commercial "sports" beverages works as a quick means of replenishing lost fluids, preventing heat stress, and obtaining calories in the form of fast-burning carbohydrates. You may prefer to dilute the beverage with water.

6. *Use ergogenic substances and supplements*—such as carnitine, inosine, branched-chain amino acids, eleutherococcus, TMG, DMG, gama-oryzanol, and hemoglobin superchargers, as described in other chapters in this book and in consulation with your coach and sports physician.

Be careful when eating during training and competition. People differ in their reactions to food consumed during the stress of working out and competing. Some athletes' performance capabilities suffer when they exercise for a long time without eating. Others can work out for hours with no apparent drop-off in performance.

Building and Repair Foods

Your muscles and other soft tissues are built from the amino acids found in proteins. Your skeletal framework is made up of minerals, such as calcium and phosphorus. Endurance-trained muscles have more and larger mitochondria than untrained muscle. Therefore, since all these structures—bone, muscle, and mitochondria—have a protein framework, it's obvious that training increases your requirements for protein.

Also, protein can provide 5–10 percent of the energy (15 percent in the glycogen-depleted athlete) used in sustained exercise. If your amino acids aren't continually replaced through your diet, you won't get enough proteins for growth and recovery from the stresses of training.

For endurance activities, you should consume about 1.5 grams of protein per kilogram of body weight, or 0.7 grams per pound—or about 10 to 15 percent of your total daily calories. Ensure that your diet provides at least that much protein. If not, supplement each meal accordingly with protein and/or amino acids. But don't eat high-protein meals immediately before or after exercise—protein synthesis is slowed during exercise. Because protein is constantly needed by the body, you need a constant intake of it, in several small feedings throughout the day.

As for meals taken before exercise, they should contain about 70 percent complex carbohydrates to ensure adequate glycogen stores, thus sparing protein for its building and repair functions. Be sure preexercise meals are low glycemic index carbohydrates

Regulatory Foods

Your body needs several substances to regulate the thousands of precise and minute chemical reactions that occur during the energy production and repair processes. For the endurance athlete, one of the most important of these substances is water.

Adequate water balance must be maintained while you exercise, especially if it's hot. Drink four to six ounces of fluid every 15 to 30 minutes. Don't wait until you feel thirsty—thirst is not an accurate indicator of your need for fluids. Chilled fluids are absorbed faster than unchilled drinks. You'll probably lose weight during exercise, most of which is water lost from sweating. Replace this water loss by drinking a pint of fluid for every pound of weight lost.

Sweating also depletes your body of sodium and other electrolytes, which you can replace by drinking a hypotonic salt beverage or water. Don't take salt tablets. Replace potassium lost in sweat by eating fruits and vegetables. Endurance athletes need extra iron and vitamin C to assure delivery of oxygen to the mitochondria for the burning of fats and carbohydrates.

Summary

We still have lots to learn about Ultimate Sports Nutrition for the endurance athlete, especially about the effects of certain food combinations and the exact vitamin requirements for the individuals. The best bet is to enhance your body's normal metabolism by taking multivitamin and mineral supplements on a daily basis and avoiding megadoses of a single nutrient. Following the above nutritional guidelines will help you get the most out of your endurance activities.

29
HYDRATION: WATER AND SPORTS DRINKS

Water is the most abundant and most important nutrient in the body. Ironically, until recently, it has been the most *neglected* nutrient in an ultimate nutritional program for athletes, due to foolish myths that water consumption causes cramps during workouts, adds weight, and inhibits performance.

Quite the opposite is true. As Dr. Michael Colgan states, "Even a small amount of dehydration reduces performance."

Water

Scientific studies conducted by Colgan and others confirm the vital role of water in peak athletic performance capabilities. Athletes and coaches have stopped shunning water and are putting it in its rightful place at the top of the list of ultimate nutrition factors.

Two-thirds of human body weight is water, contained in blood, bones, skin, and internal organs. Even dense muscle is half water, surprising as it may seem. Water is involved in nearly every bodily process, including digestion, absorption, circulation, and excretion. Water is responsible for transporting nutrients throughout the body, building new tissues, and carrying off waste products.

All foods contain water that is absorbed by the system during digestion, and fruits and vegetables contain the highest amount of chemically pure water. Tap water, ground water, and even well water usually are contaminated with environmental toxins, pesticides, industrial wastes, and heavy metals and nitrates. To obtain the purest source of drinking water, install a home purification unit or have purified, bottled water delivered to your home. Water is so important to peak athletic performance that you would be wise to make the investment in the purity and healthfulness of your water supply.

144

During strenuous exercise, the body regulates its temperature with perspiration, its natural air-conditioning system. Sweating works to keep the body cool only if the water stays on the skin. If it immediately evaporates, as occurs in the extreme dry air of desert and high mountain areas, the perspiration device fails to protect the athlete. In dry environments, the body's demand for fluid intake is increased.

The rate and amount of fluid loss during exercise depends on intensity and duration of activity and the environmental conditions of air temperature and relative humidity.

The average 150-pound adult body contains about 45 quarts of water. Fluid losses from sweating during exercise make water a critical concern to athletes. While a sedentary, 150-pound adult in a temperate climate loses about 3 quarts daily through perspiration and excretion, he can lose more than 10 quarts a day in the desert. A 150-pound marathon runner can lose even more than 10 quarts—up to 8 or 9 percent of body weight during a marathon.

Even if our 150-pound marathon runner hydrates with a total of 40 ounces of water, by drinking 5 or 6 ounces every three miles during a 24-mile race, he will have an average sweat loss of 6 ounces of water per mile. This is a fluid loss of 160 ounces, compared to water intake of only 40 ounces, leaving an alarming 120-ounce fluid deficit.

Cases of dehydration emergencies during marathon races have forced marathon officials to adopt a policy of requiring competitors to weigh in during races. Any athlete who loses 5 percent of body weight is disqualified from continuing the race—for his or her own protection, because severe, uncorrected salt depletion and dehydration are fatal.

To study the effects of dehydration on athletic performance, Dr. Fink at Ball State University's Human Performance Laboratory used a diuretic medication to deliberately dehydrate runners. The degree of dehydration was minimal—2 to 3 percent (three or four pounds) of body weight. Yet it resulted in a 3 percent reduction in performance in a 1,500-meter race and a 6 to 7 percent reduction in performance in 5,000- and 10,000-meter races.

The reason hydration is so critical to athletes is that it keeps body temperature well below the warning level of 104°F. Loss of body water through sweat occurs mostly from blood plasma, the fluid component of blood. A loss of 5 percent of body water means a loss of 10 percent of water from blood plasma, leading to reduced oxygenation of brain and muscles—crucial functions in athletic performance.

Dr. Colgan recommends a combinational strategy for assuring adequate hydration for athletic competition: make a practice of drinking copious amounts of water on a daily basis; drink water up to 20 minutes before an athletic event; and follow a carbohydrate-loading diet (because carbohydrates retain water in the system). A 150-pound marathon runner should prehydrate for an event by drinking 40 ounces of water, which, when added to the 50 ounces retained by carbohydrate loading, keeps water loss during a marathon to a safe 4 percent.

Another reason you need water is to flush out the toxic by-products of exercise, says Dr. Leroy Perry, Los Angeles sports chiropractor. "Researchers have found that, if you decrease the level of toxins in your body after exercise, you reduce the degree of soreness," he says. "But your body can't wash the toxins out of the cells as effectively if you're not drinking enough water."

Perry recommends that athletes increase their intake of water in proportion to their activity level. One-third ounce per pound of body weight if you're inactive, one-half ounce per pound if you're moderately active (walking two miles a day, for example), and two-thirds ounce per pound if you're involved in heavy training or competition.

Electrolyte Replacement Drinks

Although water is the most important element of any sports drink, you may find that water alone just doesn't hit the spot during prolonged, strenuous exercise. Marathon runners find it almost impossible to consume enough water for a long race. As one marathoner says, "The water just seems to sit there in your stomach, giving you a full, bloated feeling." Runners who chug lots of water sometimes feel drained and weak, as if their vital energy has been diluted.

The demand for a new beverage led to the development in the late 1960s of the commercial sports drink, which served to replace water and minerals (electrolytes) lost in sweating and to provide sugar for quick energy. The first to hit the market was Gatorade, in 1967, developed by Dr. Robert Cade, a kidney specialist at the University of Florida (the school's nickname: the Gators, for alligators). By having football players drink various combinations of water/carbohydrates/electrolytes, Cade came up with a formula that he eventually sold to the Stokely–Van Camp company. The new owners added sugar to the formula, and today the sweetened Gatorade outsells all other athletic drinks combined. (Not that the heavy, cloying taste is right for everyone. Many athletes can't stomach Gatorade unless they first dilute it with water.)

One recent study conducted by researchers at the University of South Carolina's Exercise Physiology Laboratory indicates that some sports drinks can significantly enhance athletic performance and are absorbed into the bloodstream as fast as water.

The study compared the performances of 19 male endurance cyclists who drank three types of fluid during 2 hours of exercise, during a 30-minute recovery period, and during an all-out exercise task that lasted about 30 minutes.

The first was a sport drink "similar in composition to Gatorade Thirst Quencher," containing moderate amounts of carbohydrate (6 percent sugar) and small amounts of electrolytes (sodium and potassium). The second drink was a low-carbohydrate drink (2.5 percent sugar) that also contained small amounts of electrolytes. The third fluid was a water placebo.

The average time needed to complete the final exercise task was significantly less with the fluid similar in composition to Gatorade than with water. The low-carbohydrate/electrolyte beverage did not significantly enhance performance over water.

Analyzing blood samples taken from each subject at regular intervals revealed no significant differences for rates of fluid entry into the blood among the three fluid types. Data from this study contradict a current opinion among some athletes, coaches, and exercise physiologists that plain water is absorbed into the body faster than any other fluid. Prior research focused only on stomach emptying, while the South Carolina research investigated how quickly fluids actually get into the bloodstream.

The small intestine absorbs fluid more rapidly from a glucose/sodium solution than from a purely saline solution. The presence of glucose stimulates sodium uptake across the small intestine, an action that significantly increases fluid absorption. This is a primary reason why sports drinks containing carbohydrates and sodium can be effective fluid replacement beverages.

The researchers said that plain, cool water always has been, and will continue to be, an effective fluid replacement beverage. However, during prolonged periods of exercise, rehydration with plain water can result in a drop of blood sugar levels and the forced mobilization of tissue energy stores—resulting in earlier fatigue and reduced endurance.

Thus, it appears that certain carbohydrate/electrolyte drinks can contribute to improved athletic performance since they supply energy and may help maintain plasma electrolyte balance. This is especially important for athletes who may dilute their blood sodium level by consuming large amounts of plain water during prolonged exercise.

Right on the heels of Gatorade, ERG (Electrolyte Replacement with Glucose) came out in 1968 in sporting goods stores. It was the only commercial drink served along the courses of the 1984 men's and women's Olympic marathons. ERG was developed by a San Diego runner and science teacher, Bill Gookin, who found Gatorade upsetting to his stomach. His goal was to invent a drink that was tolerated by the digestive system and absorbed quickly.

Gookin analyzed the perspiration of runners during a run and developed a glucose/electrolyte replacement drink that was higher in potassium, lower in sodium, and more diluted than Gatorade.

Whether or not the body actually loses electrolytes during strenuous exercise is debatable. Studies reveal conflicting results: Gookin insists electrolytes are lost and must be replaced, but Dr. David Costill of Ball State University's Human Performance Lab says no.

"We've done extensive studies on this, and all the evidence points toward the fact that you don't need electrolytes in a drink," Costill says. "We've done muscle biopsies, blood tests. We've measured electrolyte intake and output. And there's absolutely no evidence of any electrolyte deficiency."

Gookin and other marathon runners are convinced that athletes need something more than water to ward off that depleted, worn-out feeling and the soreness and stiffness that set in after a long training session. The problem with high-sugar drinks is that they tend to empty slowly from the stomach. So Gookin helped create a new drink called Max, now being test-marketed by the Coca-Cola company in two states. Max is a high-tech fluid replacement and energy drink that uses a newly developed "glucose polymer" con-

147

sisting of several glucose molecules bonded together, which permit quicker absorption in the stomach.

Another brand of drink containing this new super-carbohydrate molecule combination is Exceed, developed by Ross Laboratories of Columbus, Ohio, the original creators of glucose polymer.

In the midst of the electrolyte debate, some facts are clear: a sports drink shouldn't contain high amounts of sugar or random amounts of electrolytes, because these may retard absorption and inhibit the cooling effect of the drink.

148

Protein Drinks

Another type of sports drink is those made from protein powder. Protein drinks are especially popular among weightlifters who need more protein to build muscle mass and increase strength. The benefit of these drinks is that they provide complete protein without the high amount of fat and cholesterol associated with meat, eggs, cheese, and milk.

Most commercial protein powders are made from egg whites, soy, whey, casein, and lacto-albumin, plus added vitamins and minerals, amino acids, and carbohydrates. The added carbohydrates provide a favorable ratio of carbohydrate to protein, necessary for successful synthesis of protein in the body.

Gideon Zeidler, Ph.D., food engineer, scientist, and former director of planning and operations for Weider Health and Fitness Co., Inc. (one of the world's largest manufacturers of protein powder), believes that protein drinks are valuable not only to athletes but to everyone, because the body has a continual need for new protein in its process of renewing itself.

"Protein is something that doesn't stay in the body for very long," says Zeidler. "A muscle is composed of protein molecules, but every 120 days or so all the molecules of protein in your body are replaced by new molecules. When you consume protein, it's basically used for two purposes: to build new muscle and to replace old protein molecules.

"You're constantly replacing the molecules of protein in your body. The old molecules are broken down into amino acids; the nitrogen is taken off and converted into urea, which is excreted in the urine. The rest of the molecule is used as an energy source in the same way as sugar or fat.

"Now, if you don't consume enough protein, the body still keeps releasing the old molecules—maybe not at the same speed, but it still keeps releasing them. We see the effect of this on the bodies of people who are starving, for instance. That's why you need to keep your protein nutrition up.

"In my opinion, the issue is how well you want to perform in your sport," Zeidler says. "Do you want to be a champion, a top performer? The more you want to go in that direction, the more important this type of supplementation becomes."

149

Beer

To slake your after-workout thirst, no doubt you have chugged your fair share of beer, the traditional beverage for the dehydrated athlete. We cannot escape the connection between sports and beer—in TV commercials, sponsorship for 10Ks and marathons, and keg parties after rugby matches.

Drinking beer is considered a macho thing to do in the macho world of athletics. The main problem is that many sports heroes don't stop with one or two beers after the game—they down entire six-packs, several nights a week, week after week, year after year. Alcoholism is a major problem in sports, just as it is in society in general.

Experts say that a bottle or two after the game can help relax you and replace fluids lost in sweat. But beer is not the best choice for a drink. You're far better off chugging water.

Well, you may say, beer is 90 percent water. Sure it is—it's also 7.0 percent alcohol. That's less than the alcohol content of wine (12 percent) and hard liquor (40–50 percent), but it's still enough to knock you for a loop.

The fact is, even a small amount of alcohol—three 12-ounce bottles of beer—can impair your athletic performance. It can inhibit your reaction time, hand-eye coordination, accuracy, and balance. It lowers your heat tolerance and causes temporary changes in vision.

Furthermore, alcohol doesn't enhance metabolism or physiological functions important to exercise. If you think alcohol can improve muscular work capacity, you're mistaken. Alcohol is likely to lead to decreased performance levels.

Hold on, you argue. Beer is loaded with carbohydrates, which we athletes need in great abundance! My response is, "Big deal." Beer contains 13 grams of carbohydrates per can or bottle, one-third of the 150 calories. The other two-thirds of the calories come from alcohol, which is a worthless source of fuel for muscles because it cannot be stored as glycogen.

Beer contains many questionable ingredients that are not listed on the label, additives linked to allergic reactions in some people and even cancer in laboratory animals. Some doctors say long-term consumption of alcohol is "clearly toxic" to skeletal, muscle, and heart function and, in heavy drinkers, potentially damaging to the liver and brain.

150

If you take lots of vitamins and are a heavy alcohol drinker, you're wasting your vitamins. Alcohol blocks absorption of vitamins and washes them out of the body.

Drinking beer within 24 hours *before* an athletic event is strictly a no-no, according to several experts. Dr. David Lowenthal of Philadelphia's Hahnemann Medical College and Hospital thinks that one or two beers after a long race is "OK, relatively speaking," but shouldn't be part of the carbohydrate-loading ritual.

"Carbohydrate loaders can clearly blunt performance," says Lowenthal. "What's more, an athlete who drinks excessively and who injures himself during competition may not even perceive the pain and thus injure himself more severely. Alcohol is a semianesthetic."

And if you remain unconvinced at this point, consider this: alcohol interferes with injury recovery and the effectiveness of medication. Sports doctors report that athletes who don't drink get better results from their medication, whether it's a cold remedy or pills to reduce inflammation. No matter how you look at it, beer and other alcohol should be occasional luxury items. They don't belong in the serious athlete's diet for ultimate nutrition.

30
CARBOHYDRATE LOADING

Carbohydrate loading is an ergogenic technique for endurance athletes. It tricks your muscles into storing more fuel than they normally would.

Although carbohydrate loading has been hailed as an innovative training technique in the past few years, the discovery of carbohydrate as the preferred fuel of the body dates back several decades. In 1939 Swedish scientists demonstrated that the body burns carbohydrates before drawing upon its fat and protein.

They found that the body readily uses carbohydrates as fuel for the muscular and nervous systems with minimal waste and toxic by-products—unlike the case with proteins and fats.

The body stores carbohydrates in the form of glycogen in the muscles and liver. This glycogen helps the liver to detoxify otherwise dangerous substances. It also supplies a readily available source of glucose to maintain the essential blood sugar level.

Glycogen stored in a muscle is available for energy use for only that particular muscle, unlike glycogen stored in the liver, which is available systemically.

At rest and during low-intensity exercise, the body burns about an equal mixture of fat and carbohydrate for energy purposes. However, as work intensity increases, carbohydrates become the dominant fuel because of their quick availability.

Laboratory research has shown that at exercise intensities of less than 40 to 50 percent of your maximum oxygen consumption capability the body burns mostly fat and the degradation of stored glycogen is minimal.

The situation changes during high-intensity exercise, when carbohydrates become the sole source of energy. The activity itself is limited by the availability of glycogen as an energy source.

152

Muscle glycogen is five times more available as an energy source for intensive exercise than liver glycogen. When muscle glycogen becomes depleted, the muscle itself begins to fail and fatigue rapidly sets in. In marathon running, this dreaded phenomenon is known as "hitting the wall."

Since it is obvious that the availability of glycogen is a limiting factor in endurance athletic events, exercise physiologists have devised ways to increase glycogen storage in the body. In 1967 two Swedish exercise physiologists came up with carbohydrate loading, also call *glycogen loading*, as a method of supercompensation in glycogen through diet and exercise.

Carbohydrate loading is of no real benefit in athletic events lasting less than 60 minutes, because less activity time does not deplete glycogen levels enough to inhibit work capacity of endurance.

How To Load Up

Carbohydrate loading usually is approached by any of the following means:

1. *Consumption of high-complex-carbohydrate and high-protein foods while limiting intake of refined sugar three to four days before a competition.* This results in a glycogen level 40 to 60 percent above normal.
2. *Exercise to exhaustion for several days, followed by a carbohydrate-loading period.* This will deplete stored glycogen and then double its reserves.
3. *A combination of low carbohydrate consumption and exhaustive exercise.* The athlete eats only proteins and fats for three days, followed by eating only carbs for the next three days. On the carbo-concentration days, the athlete exercises minimally so as not to interfere with the glycogen storage process.

According to researcher David Costill, Ph.D., carbohydrate consumption in excess of 600 grams daily won't result in proportionally larger amounts of synthesized glycogen. In the first 24 hours of carbo loading, the type of carbs eaten is not of critical importance. However, after the second day, Costill suggests eating *complex* carbohydrates rather than refined or simple sugars.

Complex carbs, as we've seen, are those that contain lots of intact fiber, such as whole grains, fruits, and vegetables. An exception to this rule is pasta, which is a refined sugar but is good to ingest during carbo loading. Complex carbs tend to maintain a steady output of the hormone insulin, which activates the enzyme glycogen synthetase, essential for effective glycogen storage.

Most experts today advocate that you adopt a gradually tapering exercise program while increasing carbo consumption to about 525 grams daily. This prevents the problems associated with the low-carb period, such as fatigue, weakness, potassium loss, and muscle tissue loss.

One day prior to competition, you rest completely and consume about 55 grams of carbohydrate.

You should limit your carbohydrate-loading program to three times a year. More often than that seems to decrease its effectiveness. Costill suggests that athletes engaged in intense exercise on a daily basis consume about 70 percent of their daily calories in carbohydrates. This will maintain adequate glycogen levels in both the liver and muscles, he claims.

The Effects of Carbo Loading

Many independent studies have noted that the carbohydrate-loading technique produces these desirable effects in athletic competition:

- Muscles supercompensate in glycogen storage by *holding more than twice the normal level of muscle glycogen*. For the marathon racer, this means enough glycogen stores to run 40 miles before "hitting the wall" instead of the typical 20 to 22 miles—more than enough muscle fuel to complete a 24-mile marathon.
- Only the muscles depleted by the intense exercise session will supercompensate by doubling average glycogen levels. For the depletion technique to work, therefore, the exercise session must stress exactly the same muscles in exactly the same way as in the actual athletic event.

- Muscles store most of the glycogen in the first 24 hours after depletion.
- Muscle glycogen increases occur along with increases in vital water stores. For each gram of extra glycogen stored, the body holds another 2.7 grams of water. In competition, metabolism of the extra glycogen yields another 0.6 grams of water per gram. The doubling of muscle glycogen stores from 400 to 800 grams produces a bonus of 50 ounces of extra water for sweating during competition.

154

Some nutrition experts advocate following the depletion exercise with a low carbohydrate diet to further stimulate supercompensation. However, studies by Drs. Colgan and Costill have found that the low-carbohydrate phase is unnecessary and uncomfortable and potentially dangerous to the athlete, due to the buildup of urates in the body (uric acid causes joint stiffness associated with gout).

The supercompensation effect of carbohydrate loading is less pronounced in elite athletes—those who train about five hours a day—than in the average recreational or club athlete. This is because elite athletes are considered endurance athletes. Their long sessions of vigorous workouts deplete their glycogen stores on a daily basis. Most elite athletes follow recommended nutritional

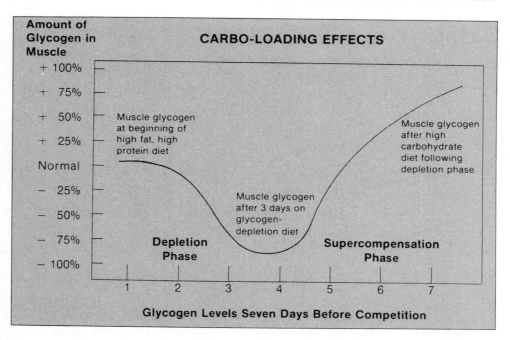

CARBO-LOADING EFFECTS

Amount of Glycogen in Muscle

+ 100%
+ 75%
+ 50%
+ 25%
Normal
− 25%
− 50%
− 75%
− 100%

Muscle glycogen at beginning of high fat, high protein diet

Muscle glycogen after high carbohydrate diet following depletion phase

Muscle glycogen after 3 days on glycogen-depletion diet

Depletion Phase

Supercompensation Phase

1 2 3 4 5 6 7

Glycogen Levels Seven Days Before Competition

programs and load up on complex carbohydrates every day. As a result, their replenished muscle glycogen stores are higher than those of recreational athletes.

Carbohydrate loading isn't for everyone. The rapid water storage it causes makes some people feel stiff and tight, resulting in decreased performance. The only way to determine if carbohydrate loading works for you is to try it—carefully!

155

31
THE PREGAME MEAL

Of all the foes that can beat you in sports, your pregame meal is one of the most formidable. The last meal you eat before game time can give you a powerful boost or cut you down before the starting signal.

By now you've got the message that you are what you eat and that ultimate nutrition for peak performance takes education and careful planning. This is especially true for the pregame meal.

"I've seen many an athlete do themselves in by a completely stupid meal, just as decisively as if by a better opponent," says Dr. Nathan Smith, professor of sports medicine at the University of Washington and author of *Food for Sport.*

"The pregame meal is too important to the success of the ensuing contest to allow it to take place willy-nilly," Smith says. "It's as important as planning the strategy for the game itself."

At the University of Washington, a group of Olympic swimmers were favored to win their events at the Pac Eight Conference swimming championships, and sure enough, they swept the preliminary events. "But between the morning semifinals and the afternoon finals, they went out to eat in style," Smith says. "They socked away steaks, french fries, and plenty of pie. At the finals, they weren't the same people. They finished poorly. One of them wasn't even able to finish his race."

The reason for their sudden shift from winners to losers: a

pregame meal heavy in fat, which requires a prodigious amount of time and energy to digest. Pregame meals of steaks, eggs, bacon, waffles, butter, and milk may be part of American sports tradition, but eating these foods is about the worst thing you can do to your body and your athletic performance.

Add stress to the situation—and stress is inherent in strenuous sports training and pregame nervous jitters—and a high-fat meal can take as long as eight hours to be completely assimilated. Fats, especially cooked fats, require more complex digestive processing than any other type of food. Fat digestion diverts blood away from the muscles and brain to the gastrointestinal tract.

This means that when you need your energy for explosive power and speed, it's not there to do the job. So your body will compensate by shifting its energy to the muscles and brain, and suddenly the digestive tract is shortchanged. Biochemical confusion ensues, potentially leading to sluggishness, fatigue, cramps, vomiting, and shortness of breath—hardly the ingredients for peak athletic performance.

Smith advises you to plan your pregame meal around those foods that have been associated with winning and peak performance in your sport. Even if a certain food doesn't really make you win, believing it does can provide the mental magic touch of confidence you need to excel.

But beware: even your most thought-out pregame meal plan can be wiped out by competition anxiety, which strikes most athletes at some point in their careers. Stress slows the digestive process and makes some athletes unable to keep down their pregame meal. Nervous tension can be controlled or redirected with various psychological methods as taught by sports psychologists and coaches.

If you're a high-strung athlete who has trouble digesting a pregame meal, try liquid meals, available from your physician. These hospital products are for patients who cannot digest solid foods, and they contain the nutrients and calories you need for energy.

Smith recommends that coaches help their teams plan the pregame meal, to be eaten together as a group. This takes care of those athletes who tend to skip meals or eat foods that undermine their game.

Here are some helpful hints for planning your pregame meal:

- Your last meal should be eaten about three hours before competing to allow for complete digestion and assimilation.

158

- Eat foods that are nongreasy, bland, nonspicy, and easily digested. These are the low glycemic index complex carbohydrates such as fruits, some vegetables, nuts, whole grains. Pancakes and waffles are OK, but go easy on the butter (fat), syrup, and jelly (simple carbohydrates). Most complex carbohydrates are high in fiber, which speeds the elimination process. To prevent this from happening at an inconvenient moment, don't consume too much dietary fiber. Try instead such complex carbs as are found in processed grains (such as pasta, white bread, pancakes, and waffles) as the main part of your pregame meal.
- The body thrives on consistency; therefore, eat foods you like and avoid those you rarely consume or aren't familiar with.
- Never skip meals. If you're dieting to lose weight, eat at least a little food, or the hunger and depression resulting from low blood sugar may interfere with your performance.
- Don't overload on protein for 12 hours prior to the game. The organic acids that protein digestion yields cannot be excreted when the body is busy in strenuous physical exercise.
- Limit intake of simple carbohydrates such as table sugar, honey, cake, cookies, and ice cream (which is also high in fat and protein). Sweets cause hypoglycemia, or unusually high levels of glucose in the blood, which quickly drop to below normal. This results in a sudden letdown of energy, devastating to you as an athlete. Excessive sugar also interferes with fluid absorption and thus can endanger a dehydrated athlete, especially in hot, humid weather.
- Avoid milk products for 24 hours prior to competition.
- Restrict your salt intake. Avoid salty foods such as table salt, monosodium glutamate, mustard, catsup, soy sauce, canned soups, bouillon cubes, relish, pickles, peanut butter, sauerkraut, dry cereals, smoked meats and fish, Worcestershire sauce, sausage, cheese, potato chips, and all salty snacks.

PART FIVE
FOOD AND RECIPE GUIDE FOR PEAK-PERFORMANCE ATHLETES

32
ALTERNATIVES TO TRADITIONAL FOODS

Tired of eating the same old things? If you have a taste for something new and exotic, check out the so-called "new age" foods. To find some of these delicious, nutritious items, you need go no farther than the produce section of your local supermarket. If your local market hasn't yet joined the new age, stop by the health food store. Alongside the carrots, lettuce, and potatoes you'll find some foods you may have never heard of before—such as hizichi, sunflower sprouts, and tempeh.

What is this, an international food bazaar? Pretty close!

These and other exotic items have made their way into the mainstream after being introduced to U.S. consumers via health food stores and ethnic markets. Some of the most outstanding values in nutritional content may be found in items that are unfamiliar to you. So let's get acquainted with some of these food products. If you're looking for "natural" foods that don't contain harmful chemicals and additives and are loaded with nutrients, you'll be glad to know about these:

Tofu

Tofu is a white, cheesy curd made from soybeans. It comes in a block packed in water in a plastic container. Slice or cube it and use it raw or cooked as a substitute for meat, cheese, eggs, or milk. A four-ounce serving of tofu contains 72 calories and yields about eight grams of usable protein and lots of vitamin B, plus potassium, calcium, and as much iron as some types of fish. The best news is that tofu is virtually fat-free, an indispensable item on a low-fat, low-calorie diet.

Tofu tastes bland and absorbs other flavors well. Use firm-style tofu in place of beef in stroganoff, cream cheese on bread, high-fat mozzarella on pizza, or half the ground beef in meat loaf.

Tempeh

Tempeh is another high-protein, all-purpose soy food, made by the natural, salt-free fermenting of soybeans, with or without the addition of grain (usually wheat or rice). It has a mild, veal-like flavor and is used as a meat substitute. With 50 percent more protein than hamburger, tempeh has only 230 calories per serving and no cholesterol. it is probably the world's richest nonmeat source of vitamin B_{12}, a nutrient that people on vegetarian diets must be especially careful to obtain.

Like tofu, tempeh lends itself to many types of quick, easy cooking: broiled, skewered and barbecued, steamed, cubed and baked, stir-fried, or cooked in stews and spaghetti sauces. You can buy tempeh ready to cook, or you can make your own with a Farm Foods kit containing beans and culture (available at health food stores).

Breads

Breads offer a variety of interesting food choices, all higher in fiber and lower in processing and calories than the usual supermarket fare. There are whole wheat pita bread, salt-free rice cakes, and flour-free Essene.

Whole wheat pita bread is the most fun: round pockets to stuff with any filling you like. Whole wheat pita contains only 160 calories per "loaf," the same as two slices of bread, and is rich in B vitamins and trace minerals and low in sodium.

Rice cakes are round, fat crackers of puffed rice, aggressively crunchy like popcorn. They are perfect for loading up with nonfat yogurt, spreads, tuna, or slices of avocado or banana—or honey or jelly, if you can afford to splurge in your diet. Containing about 34 calories per cake, they come plain or with buckwheat, millet, sesame, or corn germ, in salted, low-salt, and unsalted varieties. Next time you get the urge for potato chips or corn chips, reach for rice cakes instead. But be warned: this healthful, high-fiber snack can be addicting, so don't be surprised if you find yourself demolishing half a bag at one sitting!

Essene bread, or wayfarer's bread, comes in a dense, heavy, round loaf. It is the most healthful of the new-age breads (actually it dates from biblical times), because it contains only water and sprouted grains—wheat or rye, plus a combination with seeds and fruits. It is baked at a very low temperature to conserve vitamins and minerals.

163

Tahini

This sesame seed paste, imported from the Middle East, is a spread that can replace peanut butter. Tahini is rich in calcium and essential fatty acids. Spread it on breads, crackers, or rice cakes or make a salad dressing by diluting it with lemon juice and Oriental rice vinegar. Eat it sparingly, because spreads made from nuts and seeds are high in fat.

Miso

Miso is a soybean product, mildly salty and rich in B vitamins, used as a flavoring in place of A-1 Sauce and in soups and gravies. One of the all-time, classic "health" foods, miso contains digestive enzymes that help you assimilate your food. Miso soup is the traditional Oriental equivalent of the Western world's chicken soup. Dilute and drink it as a coffee substitute. Try mixing miso with tahini for a great sandwich spread.

Oriental Noodles

This Eastern form of pasta is higher in protein than conventional noodles. Instead of spaghetti, use udon, which is a flat, light-textured noodle available made of whole wheat. Or make soups with soba—thin, round, hearty noodles fortified with buckwheat. Ramen is a soup noodle made with 80 percent whole wheat flour and 20 percent unbleached white wheat flour. Another good choice for pasta is soy-fortified macaroni (e.g., Superoni) which provides high-quality protein and can help lower blood pressure and cholesterol.

Sea Vegetables

These, including seaweeds from the Orient, are used in place of lettuce and salad greens. Available in about eight varieties, sea vegetables contain more vitamin A, B, and C than romaine lettuce or kale and more potassium than bananas or nuts. Hizichi resembles shredded black cabbage but cooks like spaghetti. Try it in everything from soups to stir-fried dishes—hizichi has more calcium than cottage cheese and 10 times the iron of spinach. Nori and rame are other sea vegetables high in vitamins and minerals that are easy to cook. Both are excellent as soup additives or when eaten separately.

Sprouts

Sprouts now are available in many varieties besides mung beans and alfalfa. Wheat sprouts are round and seedlike. They are low-calorie, high-fiber, sweet, and chewy—tasty when stir-fried or sprinled over salad, yogurt, or soybean frozen dessert. Also try sprouted chick-peas (garbanzo beans), pumpkin seeds, adzuki beans, and sunflower seeds.

Sweet Acidophilus Milk

This milk was developed by the food science department at North Carolina State University in a tasty formula containing healthy organisms that implant themselves in your gastrointestinal tract to aid digestion. Unlike *Lactobacillus bulgaricus*, the strain used in most common brands of fermented milk, *Lactobacillu acidophilus* is not destroyed by stomach acids. Commercially, this strain is available in the brand names Erivan, Sundance, and Brown Cow Farm. Sweet acidophilus milk yields 10 times the calcium found in meat or fish. Eating yogurt made with acidophilus lowers the levels of certain cancer-causing enzymes in the intestines.

Soybean Ice Creams

These alternatives are made without eggs, milk, or additives, making them virtually free of fat and cholesterol and a perfect frozen dessert for people who are allergic to milk and dairy products. Popular brand names are Tofutti and Ice Dream.

Snack Chips

There are now varieties without salt, sugar, or unsaturated fats. Bye-bye, potato chips: welcome, banana chips! And let's not overlook the new, baked (not fried) chips made from mushrooms, brown rice, carrots, yogurt, and green onions.

Sweeteners

Sweeteners are made from many substances besides sugar. There are dehydrated maple syrup granules, made by Vermont Country Maple, which is 60 percent as sweet as sugar and contains all the nutrients sugar lacks, such as calcium and magnesium, with none of the additives. Barley malt extract comes in syrup or granules and is 25 percent as sweet as honey. Rice honey is made from whole bran and barley rice in a low-temperature cooking process that saves the minerals and B vitamins from destruction.

So you see, your quest for ultimate nutrition will introduce you to some fantastic new foods from faraway places. There is a lot to choose from besides the traditional, low-fiber, high-fat American diet.

33
BREAKFASTS OF CHAMPIONS

Spicy Apples and Sausages

Serve with hot oatmeal topped with milk, brown sugar, and ground cinnamon; plain low-fat yogurt with strawberries; and hot tea.

- 1 tablespoon reduced-calorie margarine
- 2 small apples, cored and sliced
- ½ cup diced onion
- 6 ounces smoked sausages, cut into ¼-inch-thick slices
- 1 teaspoon firmly packed brown sugar
- ⅛ teaspoon each dried sage leaves, ground cloves, and ground cinnamon

In 8-inch nonstick skillet, heat margarine until hot and bubbly; add apples and onion and sauté until golden. Add remaining ingredients and stir to combine; cover and let simmer until apples are soft, about 5 minutes. Serve with toast (not included in nutritional evaluation).

Serves 2

Nutritive values per serving:	CAL	PRO (gm)	FAT (gm)	CHO (gm)
	386	10	28	24

Cornmeal Pancakes

Serve with orange juice with a mint sprig, broiled Canadian bacon, and cinnamon-spiced coffee.

⅓ cup (3 ounces) cornmeal
¼ teaspoon baking soda
¼ teaspoon salt
½ cup buttermilk
1 egg
3 tablespoons reduced-calorie maple syrup

168

Sift together dry ingredients onto a sheet of waxed paper or a paper plate. Set aside. In a medium bowl, beat together milk and egg; gradually stir in cornmeal mixture, stirring until smooth.

Spray 10-inch skillet with nonstick cooking spray and heat. Make 4 pancakes by dropping half the batter into pan by heaping tablespoonsful. Cook until edges are browned and bubbles appear on surface. Turn pancakes over and cook until browned on other side. Place pancakes on serving platter and keep warm. Repeat procedure with second half of batter. Serve each portion with about 2 teaspoons syrup.

Serves 4, 2 pancakes each

Nutritive values per serving:				
	CAL	PRO (gm)	FAT (gm)	CHO (gm)
	129	4	2	23

Sautéed Peppered Liver

Serve with grapefruit juice, a bran muffin and butter, a dish of plain nonfat yogurt, and hot coffee.

2 teaspoons vegetable oil
½ cup sliced onion
½ cup red bell pepper strips
1 garlic clove, minced
10 ounces beef or calf liver, cut into thin strips
2 tablespoons all-purpose flour
1 tablespoon teriyaki sauce
1 tablespoon catsup
Dash freshly ground pepper
⅓ cup water

In 10-inch skillet, heat oil over medium heat. Add onion, red pepper, and garlic and sauté until vegetables are tender. Add liver and sauté until meat is no longer red, about 3 minutes (do not overcook). Sprinkle mixture with flour, then stir in teriyaki sauce, catsup, and pepper. Gradually add water and, stirring constantly, bring to a boil. Reduce heat to low and cook, stirring, for 1 to 2 minutes.

Serves 2

Nutritive values per serving:

CAL	PRO (gm)	FAT (gm)	CHO (gm)
296	29	10	20

Griddle Cakes

Serve with orange and grapefruit sections, egg, and hot cocoa.

- ⅓ cup plus 2 teaspoons each whole wheat flour and all-purpose flour
- 1 teaspoon sugar
- ¾ teaspoon double-acting baking powder
  Dash each salt and ground cinnamon
- ½ cup evaporated skim milk
- ⅓ cup cottage cheese
- 1 egg

In medium mixing bowl, sift together flours, sugar, baking powder, salt, and cinnamon. In blender, combine milk, cheese, and egg and blend until smooth; stir into dry ingredients, mixing thoroughly.

Spray 9- or 10-inch nonstick skillet or griddle with nonstick cooking spray and heat over medium-high heat; using half of the batter, make 4 cakes by dropping batter by heaping tablespoonsful into skillet or onto griddle. Cook until bottom is browned and bubbles appear on surface. Turn cakes over and cook until other side is browned. Remove to serving platter and keep warm. Using remaining batter, repeat procedure, spraying pan with cooking spray and making 4 more cakes.

Serves 4, 2 griddle cakes each

Nutritive values per serving:

CAL	PRO (gm)	FAT (gm)	CHO (gm)
140	9	2	22

Bran 'n' Blueberry Muffins

Serve with orange juice, omelet, melon slices, and hot coffee or tea.

- 1¼ cups whole wheat flour
- ¾ cup wheat germ
- 1½ cups bran flakes
- 2 teaspoons baking powder
- 1 teaspoon baking soda
- ¼ teaspoon ground cinnamon
- 1 cup blueberries
- 1 cup shredded apple
- ⅓ cup orange juice concentrate
- ¾ cup evaporated skim milk
- 3 egg whites

Mix all dry ingredients and add blueberries and apple. Combine all liquid ingredients. Add to flour mixture and blend well. Spray muffin tin with nonstick vegetable spray. Fill each tin two-thirds full with mixture. Bake at 350°F for 30 to 35 minutes, until tops turn golden brown.

Serves 24 (1 muffin per serving)

Nutritive values per serving:	CAL	PRO (gm)	FAT (gm)	CHO (gm)
	102	4	1	21

Potato Omelet

Serve with buttermilk biscuits, applesauce with raisins, orange slices, and hot coffee or tea.

- 4 eggs
  Dash each salt, ground nutmeg, and freshly ground pepper
- 1 tablespoon vegetable oil
- ½ cup diced onion
- 2 ounces Canadian-style bacon, diced
- 6 ounces potatoes, peeled, cooked, and cut into ⅛-inch-thick slices

In medium bowl, beat eggs with salt, nutmeg, and pepper; set aside. In 8-inch nonstick skillet, heat oil, add onion and bacon, and sauté over high heat until onion turns clear. Add potato slices and cook, turning, until browned on all sides. Gently shake pan until potato slices lie flat in bottom of skillet and do not overlap. Stir egg mixture, then pour over potatoes. Cover skillet and cook over low heat until eggs are set and firm, about 5 minutes.

Serves 2

171

Nutritive values per serving:

CAL	PRO (gm)	FAT (gm)	CHO (gm)
334	20	20	18

Rice-Raisin Pudding

Serve with papaya juice, whole wheat toast and jelly, sliced bananas, and hot coffee.

- 1 cup skim milk
- ¾ ounce uncooked regular long-grain rice
- 1½ teaspoons sugar
- Dash salt
- 1 egg
- 2 tablespoons raisins
- ½ teaspoon vanilla extract
- Dash ground cinnamon

In a 1-quart saucepan, combine milk, rice, sugar, and salt and bring to a boil. Reduce heat to low, cover, and let simmer, stirring occasionally, until rice is tender and mixture is creamy, 15 to 20 minutes.

In a small bowl, beat egg; add ¼ cup hot rice mixture and stir to combine. Slowly stir egg mixture into saucepan and cook over low heat, stirring constantly, until pudding thickens (do not overcook). Stir in raisins and vanilla. Transfer to serving bowl and sprinkle with cinnamon. Serve warm or cover and refrigerate until chilled.

Serves 2

Nutritive values per serving:

CAL	PRO (gm)	FAT (gm)	CHO (gm)
164	8	3	25

Oatmeal Deluxe

Serve with orange juice, egg, and hot cocoa.

- 1½ cups water
- 1 tablespoon orange juice concentrate
- ¼ cup raisins
- 1 cup oatmeal
- Dash ground cinnamon
- ½ banana, halved and sliced
- 1 apple, peeled and diced

Put water, orange juice concentrate, and raisins in small saucepan. Bring to a boil and add oatmeal. Turn off heat and stir constantly. Add cinnamon and fruit. Leave over still-warm burner for about 1 minute, stirring constantly. Remove from heat and serve hot. Top with plain nonfat yogurt (not included in nutritional evaluation).

Serves 2

Nutritive values per serving:	CAL	PRO (gm)	FAT (gm)	CHO (gm)
	228	4.3	2.3	58

Steamed Acorn Squash

Serve with pineapple slices, broiled ham steak, bran muffins, and hot coffee or tea.

- 1 acorn squash, halved and seeded
- 2 tablespoons raisins
- 2 teaspoons margarine, melted
- 2 teaspoons maple syrup
- ½ teaspoon firmly packed brown sugar
- ½ teaspoon ground cinnamon
- ¼ teaspoon ground nutmeg

Slice about ⅛ inch off bottom of each squash half so that halves will stand flat. Fill a large soup pot with 2 inches of water and bring to a boil. Place squash halves in a steamer tray and place in pot; cover and let steam until squash is tender but not mushy. Remove and place cut side up on serving plates. In a small bowl, combine remaining ingredients and brush or pour sauce over each half.

Serves 2

Nutritive values per serving:

CAL	PRO (gm)	FAT (gm)	CHO (gm)
141	2	4	28

Cheese-Stuffed Potatoes

Serve with grapefruit juice, broiled ham slices, and a bowl of strawberries.

- 2 medium potatoes, baked
- 4 tablespoons low-fat cottage cheese
- 4 tablespoons grated cheddar cheese
- 4 tablespoons plain low-fat yogurt
- 1 teaspoon dried dill weed
- 3 tablespoons chopped green onion
  Dash paprika

Preheat oven to 350°F. Cut potatoes in half and carefully spoon out center. Blend cheeses, yogurt, and dill weed until smooth. Add green onion. Spoon mixture into potato shells and sprinkle with paprika. Bake for 15 to 20 minutes.

Serves 4

Nutritive values per serving:

CAL	PRO (gm)	FAT (gm)	CHO (gm)
98	5.3	2.7	12.8

34
WEIGHT-LOSS RECIPES

Hibiscus Float

¾ cup unsweetened pineapple juice
½ medium papaya, seeded, peeled, and chunked
½ persimmon, peeled and sliced
2 ounces nonfat yogurt
1 tablespoon fresh lime juice
2–3 ice cubes
   Honey to taste
4 ounces carbonated water

Mix all ingredients except carbonated water in blender or food processor. When drink is a thick, creamy consistency, pour into a glass and add carbonated water.

Serves 1

Nutritive values per serving:	CAL	PRO (gm)	FAT (gm)	CHO (gm)
	241	5	1	50

Kona Coffee Whip

1 cup nonfat milk
¾ cup brewed Kona coffee
½ banana, sliced
1 egg white
1 heaping tablespoon raw wheat germ
2 tablespoons protein powder
2–3 ice cubes
Honey or pure maple syrup to taste

Mix ingredients in a blender until thick and creamy.

Serves 1

Nutritive values per serving:

	CAL	PRO (gm)	FAT (gm)	CHO (gm)
	291	27	1	44

Volcano Sunrise

¾ cup coconut milk, chilled
¾ cup fresh carrot juice, chilled
¾ cup fresh pineapple chunks
¼ cup grated coconut, unsweetened
1 heaping tablespoon nonfat powdered milk
3–4 ice cubes
Honey to taste

Combine all ingredients in blender and drink.

Serves 1

Nutritive values per serving:

	CAL	PRO (gm)	FAT (gm)	CHO (gm)
	263	6	12	40

Mango Mint Frappé

¾ cup fresh orange juice, chilled
1 medium mango, peeled, pitted, and chunked
1 medium nectarine, peeled, pitted, and chunked
2–3 fresh mint leaves
3–4 ice cubes
Honey to taste

Combine all ingredients in blender and drink.

Serves 1

Nutritive values per serving:

	CAL	PRO (gm)	FAT (gm)	CHO (gm)
	272	10	2	64

177

Fish Stock

Use this stock for the following seafood stew recipes.

- 1 pound fish trimmings (heads, tails, bones, shells (from shellfish)
- 1 small onion, chopped
- ½ cup chopped shallots
- 1 carrot, sliced
- 1 stalk celery, sliced
- 2 tablespoons chopped fresh parsley
- ½ bay leaf
- ¼ teaspoon dried thyme
- ¼ teaspoon dried marjoram
- 2 cloves
- 4 peppercorns
- ⅓ teaspoon grated lemon zest
- 1 quart water
- 2 tablespoons butter
- 1 cup dry white wine

Place all ingredients except wine in a large kettle. Bring to a boil, then simmer about 15 minutes. Skim off any scum that comes to the surface. Add wine and simmer, covered, another 15 minutes. Strain through a colander.

Mussel Ratatouille

3 dozen mussels
3 cups water
3 shallots, minced
1 clove fresh garlic, minced
1 small green pepper, diced
1 tablespoon olive oil
3 cups Fish Stock
2 cups eggplant, peeled and cubed
2 medium zucchini, sliced
2 cups peeled and chopped tomatoes
2 tablespoons minced fresh parsley
½ teaspoon Italian seasoning
¼ cup Marsala wine
Salt and freshly ground pepper to taste

Scrub and debeard mussels. Steam them in water for 5 minutes. When mussel shells open, remove meat and discard shells. Sauté shallots, garlic, and green pepper in olive oil until tender. Add stock, vegetables, and seasoning and cook over medium heat until vegetables are semitender. Add wine and mussels. Reduce heat and simmer several more minutes.

Serves 4

Nutritive values per serving:

	CAL	PRO (gm)	FAT (gm)	CHO (gm)
	197	57	5	18

Scallop Curry

1 medium onion, chopped
1 teaspoon sesame oil
2 cups Fish Stock
1 tablespoon crushed sesame seeds
2 tablespoons curry powder
2 bay leaves
1 cup coconut milk (see note below)
3 dozen scallops, shucked and rinsed
Salt to taste
½ cup freshly grated coconut

Sauté onion in sesame oil until clear. Add stock and spices and simmer slowly for 30 minutes. Remove bay leaves, add coconut milk, and cook over high heat about 5 minutes, stirring constantly. Add scallops and simmer briefly, until they are opaque. Add salt to taste and sprinkle with freshly grated coconut.

Note: To make coconut milk, pour ½ cup hot water over 1 cup freshly grated coconut. Let sit 10 minutes, then press liquid through a cheesecloth-lined sieve.

179

Serves 4

Nutritive values per serving:

CAL	PRO (gm)	FAT (gm)	CHO (gm)
271	38	5	11

Beef Heart Meat Loaf

1 pound ground beef heart
2 eggs, beaten
½ cup wheat germ
¼ cup evaporated skim milk
½ cup grated carrots
½ cup chopped onion
1 teaspoon dried sage
1 clove garlic, minced
½ teaspoon dried marjoram
¼ teaspoon freshly ground black pepper
Salt to taste

Combine all ingredients in a large bowl and mix well. Shape into a loaf and place in a loaf pan coated with vegetable spray, such as Pam. Bake at 375°F for 45 minutes.

Serves 4

Nutritive values per serving:

CAL	PRO (gm)	FAT (gm)	CHO (gm)
240	27.7	8.5	14.4

Tofu-Zucchini Stew

    1 pound tofu, solid block preferred
   ¼ cup apple juice
    1 tablespoon tamari
   12 water chestnuts, quartered
    1 medium red onion, chopped
    1 ½-inch-diameter leek, chopped
    1 teaspoon herbal seasoning
    2 cups sliced zucchini
    2 medium tomatoes, chopped
      Sea salt to taste
      Freshly ground pepper (optional)
    6 ounces whole wheat or spinach noodles, cooked

Dice tofu in ½-inch squares and sauté in mixture of apple juice and tamari. Add water chestnuts, onion, leek, herbal seasoning, and zucchini. Cook at low heat for 15 minutes, adding spring water as needed for cooking liquid, but keep it to a minimum. Add tomatoes, sea salt, and pepper if desired and continue to simmer another 10 to 15 minutes. Serve over the noodles or mix together and bake at 350°F for 30 minutes to achieve a casserole effect.

Serves 4

Nutritive values per serving:

CAL	PRO (gm)	FAT (gm)	CHO (gm)
226	14	6	32

Curried Chicken and Potatoes

    2 large potatoes, baked
   ½ cup chicken broth
   ½ cup nonfat milk
    1 cup ricotta cheese
    4 ounces chicken meat, cooked and chopped
      Curry powder

While potatoes are baking, combine chicken broth and nonfat milk in a saucepan over medium heat—do not boil. When broth mixture is hot, slowly stir in ricotta cheese until mixture is smooth. When potatoes are tender, slice or dice them with skins in a medium-sized bowl. Add chicken and stir in broth/milk/cheese mixture. Mix well so potatoes are uniformly covered and moistened with liquid. Add more nonfat milk if the mixture is too dry. Season with curry powder to taste or serve curry powder at the table to please individual tastes.

Serves 2

Nutritive values per serving:

CAL	PRO (gm)	FAT (gm)	CHO (gm)
430	37	5	41

Middle Eastern Chicken and Vegetables

1	pound chicken nuggets (cut-up white meat)
1½	pounds onions, sliced (about 6 cups)
2	tablespoons corn oil
½	teaspoon ground coriander
¼	teaspoon ground cinnamon
½	teaspoon turmeric
1	teaspoon ground cumin
	Freshly ground black pepper to taste
3	tomatoes
4	ounces red pepper, sliced (slightly less than 1 cup)
3	ounces carrots, sliced or cut into sticks (heaping ½ cup)
1	tablespoon coarsely grated fresh ginger
1	teaspoon minced garlic in vegetable oil
1	cup chicken stock

Wash and dry chicken. Cut onions into large dice and sauté with chicken in hot corn oil. As chicken cooks, add coriander, cinnamon, turmeric, cumin, and pepper. Cook until chicken is white on all sides. Cut tomatoes into medium chunks. Cut red pepper slices into medium dice. Cut carrots into large dice. Add ginger, garlic, stock, and vegetables to chicken. Cover and cook 12 to 15 minutes.

Serves 3 or 4

Nutritive values per serving:

CAL	PRO (gm)	FAT (gm)	CHO (gm)
418	42	15.5	29

Oriental Beef Heart

1 tablespoon sesame oil
1 pound beef heart, sliced thin across grain and cut into 1½-inch-long strips
2 tablespoons soy sauce
1 head bok choy (Chinese cabbage)
1 cup sliced fresh mushrooms
1 cup chopped onion
1 8-ounce can sliced water chestnuts
1 tablespoon whole wheat flour, dissolved in 2 tablespoons water

Heat oil in a wok or large saucepan to about 300°F. Add beef heart; stir-fry until heart starts to lose its redness. Add the next five ingredients; stir-fry 2 minutes. Add flour mixture; stir-fry until sauce begins to thicken. Serve immediately.

Serves 4

Nutritive values per serving:

	CAL	PRO (gm)	FAT (gm)	CHO (gm)
	263	23.7	8.3	25

Fresh Tuna with Capers and Lemon

¾ pound fresh tuna
Vegetable oil
½ lemon with skin
2 teaspoons drained capers

Brush fish with vegetable oil and broil about 3 inches from source of heat on both sides until it is opaque and firm to the touch, 10 to 15 minutes, depending on thickness of fish. Follow the Canadian rule for cooking fish: measure fish at thickest part and allow 10 minutes per inch.

Dice lemon, leaving peel on, and mix with capers. When fish is cooked, sprinkle capers and lemon over fish and serve.

Serves 2

Nutritive values per serving:

	CAL	PRO (gm)	FAT (gm)	CHO (gm)
	286	40	11	3.2

Poached Salmon with Balsamic Vinegar and Tomato Relish

Relish

⅛ cup balsamic vinegar (see note below)
2 ripe tomatoes, peeled, seeded, and diced fine
2 shallots, diced fine
1 small lemon

Salmon

1½ cups equal parts fresh fennel, carrots, celery, and onion, diced fine or sliced (see note below)
2 cloves garlic, diced
1 bay leaf
¼ cup white wine vinegar
4 peppercorns
5 cups water
12 ounces fresh salmon fillets

Combine relish ingredients and let stand for 10 minutes.

Make a court bouillon by combining all remaining ingredients except salmon, bringing to a boil and cooking slowly for about 20 minutes. Add the salmon fillets and poach until barely cooked through—3 to 8 minutes, depending on thickness. Remove fillets, drain, and serve covered with tomato relish. Garnish with grilled new potatoes studded with garlic and fresh basil.

Note: If balsamic vinegar is unavailable, substitute a mixture of ⅛ cup red wine vinegar and 1 tablespoon honey. If dried fennel seed is substituted for fresh, use just a pinch and increase other vegetables to make 1½ cups total.

Serves 4

Nutritive values per serving:	CAL	PRO (gm)	FAT (gm)	CHO (gm)
	156	19	3	0

Stuffed Baked Apples

1 red apple
1 tablespoon each raisins and chopped walnuts
1 teaspoon butter
   Dash each ground cinnamon and ground nutmeg

184

Core and peel apple to one-half inch from the bottom. Stuff apple with raisins, walnuts, and butter. Sprinkle with cinnamon and nutmeg. Place apple in a shallow pan with one-fourth inch of water. Cover and bake at 400°F 45 to 50 minutes.

Variations
Other tasty fillings for the apples:
    Sunflower seeds and honey with melted cheddar cheese on top
    Cottage cheese, sprinkled with cinnamon
    Chopped bananas, peaches, or apricots, sprinkled with flaked
        coconut

Serves 1

Nutritive values per 1-apple serving:	CAL	PRO (gm)	FAT (gm)	CHO (gm)
	250	3	14	35

35
WEIGHT-GAIN RECIPES

No-Pasta Italian Cuisine
Basic Marinara Sauce

24 ounces tomato puree (3 8-ounce cans)
 1 clove garlic, minced
 1 teaspoon dried basil
 1 tablespoon olive oil
 1 tablespoon grated Parmesan or Romano cheese
 1 medium sprig fresh parsley, minced
   Salt and freshly ground pepper to taste

Simmer all ingredients in saucepan 1 hour on medium heat. Dilute with water if sauce becomes too thick during cooking. Use with the Zucchini and Meatballs recipe (page 186).

Makes about 3 cups

Zucchini and Meatballs

¾ pound ground sirloin
1 egg
½ cup grated carrot
1 medium onion, chopped fine
1 clove garlic, minced
¼ teaspoon Italian spices
   Salt and freshly ground pepper to taste
3 cups Basic Marinara Sauce
6 medium zucchini

Combine all ingredients except zucchini, and form meatballs. Brown meatballs evenly over medium heat for about 5 minutes in a nonstick frying pan. Add Basic Marinara Sauce and simmer for 1 hour more. Cut 6 medium zucchini lengthwise into thin strips (or shred in a food processor). Drop zucchini into boiling water for 3–4 minutes and remove. Ladle marinara sauce with meatballs over zucchini on individual plates and serve hot.

Serves 6

Nutritive values per serving:

	CAL	PRO (gm)	FAT (gm)	CHO (gm)
	575	25	20	55

Turkey Cannelloni

8 ounces part-skim ricotta cheese
1 egg, beaten
1 cup loosely packed finely chopped parsley
   Salt to taste
8 2-ounce slices turkey breast
16 ounces Basic Marinara Sauce
8 1-ounce slices mozzarella cheese
   Grated Parmesan cheese

In a bowl, mix ricotta, egg, parsley (save a tablespoon for garnish), and salt. Lay each slice of turkey out flat, putting 2 tablespoons of ricotta filling in the center of the slice. Then roll it up, securing with a toothpick. Repeat with each slice of turkey and place rolls opening side down on a baking sheet or in a large dish. Spoon an ample amount of marinara sauce over each roll and top with a slice of mozzarella cheese. Bake at 325°F for 25 minutes. Sprinkle with reserved parsley and parmesan cheese.

Serves 4

Nutritive values per serving:

CAL	PRO (gm)	FAT (gm)	CHO (gm)
500	49	21	25

Beef and Veal
Eggplant-Mushroom Moussaka

1½ pounds lean ground beef
2 onions, diced
1 cup sliced mushrooms
1 6-ounce can tomato paste
1 cup water
¾ cup dry white wine
2 tablespoons chopped fresh parsley
⅓ teaspoon ground cinnamon
⅛ teaspoon ground nutmeg
⅛ teaspoon freshly ground pepper
⅓ cup whole wheat bread crumbs
1 eggplant, peeled and sliced thin
   Ground nutmeg

Brown meat in a nonstick skillet and drain fat. Add onions, mushrooms, tomato paste, water, wine, parsley, cinnamon, nutmeg, and pepper. Cover and simmer for 40 minutes. Stir in bread crumbs. Remove mixture to medium-sized nonstick baking dish and add layer of eggplant slices. Continue to layer meat mixture with eggplant until used up. Sprinkle with a small amount of additional nutmeg and bake in a 350°F oven for 45 minutes.

Serves 4

Nutritive values per serving:

CAL	PRO (gm)	FAT (gm)	CHO (gm)
443	39	18	23

Beef and Vegetable Shish Kebabs

4 ounces lean sirloin tip steak, cut into 1-inch squares, fat trimmed off
4 cherry tomatoes
½ green pepper, cut into 1-inch cubes
4 mushroom caps
1 8-ounce can boiled white onions
1 slice fresh pineapple, cut into 1-inch chunks
1 teaspoon cider vinegar
¼ cup freshly squeezed tomato juice
¼ teaspoon dry mustard
⅛ teaspoon garlic powder
Dash freshly ground pepper

Thread meat, tomatoes, green pepper, mushroom caps, onions, and pineapple alternately onto shish kebab skewers. Heat vinegar, tomato juice, mustard, garlic powder, and pepper in a small pot. Place skewers in broiler about 3 inches away from heat and brush tomato juice mixture on meat and vegetables. Broil for 7 minutes, turning and brushing with mixture every 1½ minutes.

Serves 1

Nutritive values per serving:

CAL	PRO (gm)	FAT (gm)	CHO (gm)
427	22	28	22

Stuffed Green Peppers

2 large green peppers
1 cup water
½ pound lean ground beef
1 cup dry whole wheat bread crumbs
1 tablespoon chopped onion
¼ teaspoon dried oregano
¼ teaspoon dried basil
¼ teaspoon freshly ground pepper
1 8-ounce can tomato sauce

Cut tops off green peppers and remove seeds and pith. Wash. Bring water to boil. Stand peppers upright in water and cook 5 minutes. Drain water. Mix remaining ingredients and stuff peppers with them. Stand peppers upright in nonstick baking pan and bake, covered, in a 325°F oven for 45 minutes. Uncover and bake for 5 minutes.

Serves 2

Nutritive values per serving:

CAL	PRO (gm)	FAT (gm)	CHO (gm)
469	38	15	71

Veal Chops Mozzarella

2 8-ounce veal chops
2 ounces low-fat mozzarella cheese, sliced thin
¼ cup whole wheat flour
   Pinch freshly ground pepper
2 egg whites, slightly beaten
2 cups whole wheat bread crumbs
½ cup tomato juice
   Dash freshly ground white pepper
   Dash dry parsley flakes

Cut a pocket in each veal chop by cutting to the bone. Pound chops until they are ½ inch thick, then place cheese in the pockets and secure with a toothpick. Combine flour and pinch of pepper and coat chops. Dip chops in egg whites and then bread crumbs. Repeat. Sauté chops in tomato juice for 7 minutes on each side. Season with white pepper and parsley flakes and serve.

Serves 2

Nutritive values per serving:

CAL	PRO (gm)	FAT (gm)	CHO (gm)
922	59	35	90

Chicken and Fish
Chicken Stew

2 pounds chicken pieces, skinned
1 onion, sliced thin
2 large sprigs fresh dill
1 sprig fresh parsley
2 tomatoes, peeled and diced
4 carrots, scraped and cut into chunks
4 potatoes, peeled and quartered
4 celery stalks, cut into chunks
1 cup dry white wine
2 tablespoons fresh lemon juice
1 bay leaf
$\frac{1}{4}$ teaspoon freshly ground pepper

Place chicken in Dutch oven and add onion, dill, and parsley. Arrange tomatoes, carrots, potatoes, and celery around the chicken and add wine, lemon juice, bay leaf, and pepper. Cover and bake in a 350°F oven for 1½ hours. Chill and skim excess fat. Reheat and serve.

Serves 4

Nutritive values per serving:

	CAL	PRO (gm)	FAT (gm)	CHO (gm)
	438	43	9	45

Exotic Chicken and Fruit

4 pounds frying chicken pieces, skinned
2 teaspoons garlic powder
$\frac{1}{8}$ teaspoon freshly ground pepper
8 dried figs, halved
1 apple, cored and sliced into rings
$\frac{1}{2}$ cup dried apricots
1 cup raisins
1 cup water
1 cup dry white wine
$\frac{1}{8}$ cup natural honey
2 teaspoons hot dry mustard
$\frac{1}{2}$ teaspoon dried rosemary

Sprinkle chicken with garlic powder and pepper. Bake in a 350°F oven for 45 minutes in a medium nonstick pan. Combine figs, apple, apricots, raisins, water, wine, honey, mustard, and rosemary. Boil fruit mixture for 30 minutes. Pour fruit mixture over chicken. Use a baster to lift juices from baking pan and spread over chicken and fruit. Bake in 400°F oven for 15 minutes. Serve over rice. (Rice not included in nutritional calculations.)

Serves 4

Nutritive values per serving:

CAL	PRO (gm)	FAT (gm)	CHO (gm)
603	62	23	56

Salmon Salad with Artichokes

1½ pounds cooked salmon
    Salmon Dressing (recipe follows)
1 head romaine lettuce
1 pound asparagus, cooked
1 pound new potatoes, cooked and cut into chunks
1 cup sliced carrots
2 tomatoes, cut into wedges
1 6-ounce jar artichoke hearts, halved
2 tablespoons grated Romano cheese

Break cooked salmon into large chunks and set aside. Make Salmon Dressing (recipe follows) and set aside. Line platter with romaine lettuce leaves. Place salmon in center and surround with asparagus, potatoes, carrots, tomatoes, and artichoke hearts. Top with Romano cheese and dressing.

Serves 4

Nutritive values per serving:

CAL	PRO (gm)	FAT (gm)	CHO (gm)
566	47	24	41

Salmon Dressing

3 tablespoons olive oil
½ cup Dijon mustard
2 cloves garlic, crushed
3 tablespoons fresh lemon juice
¼ teaspoon dried basil
1½ tablespoons chopped fresh parsley
1 tablespoon capers
Dash freshly ground pepper

Combine all ingredients in a tightly covered container and shake well. Chill and serve or serve room temperature over Salmon Salad with Artichokes.

Serves 4

Nutritive values per serving:

	CAL	PRO (gm)	FAT (gm)	CHO (gm)
	95	0.1	10.5	0.4

192

36
CARBO-LOADING RECIPES

French Toast

1 egg, beaten
1 tablespoon bran
¼ cup nonfat milk
⅛ teaspoon coconut extract
2 slices whole wheat bread

Topping
¼ cup crushed pineapple
½ teaspoon cornstarch
¼ banana, sliced
1 tablespoon syrup

Combine egg, bran, milk, and extract and dip bread in egg mixture. Preheat nonstick pan and cook bread in it on medium heat until golden brown. For topping, mix crushed pineapple with cornstarch and simmer all topping ingredients in small pan until thickened. Serve topping on French toast.

Serves 1

Nutritive values per serving:	CAL	PRO (gm)	FAT (gm)	CHO (gm)
	278	12	6	44

Millet Marvel

Dry

$\frac{1}{3}$ cup short-grain brown rice
$\frac{1}{3}$ cup buckwheat
$\frac{1}{3}$ cup millet
$\frac{1}{3}$ cup barley flakes
$\frac{1}{4}$ cup bran

194

Wet

1 large banana
2 tablespoons honey
2 tablespoons barley malt

Pour 2 cups of water into saucepan, add dry ingredients, and stir. Simmer about 1 hour over low heat. Cereal will thicken, so add more water and keep stirring. After cereal has simmered about 20 minutes, mix wet ingredients by crushing banana in a small bowl and adding honey and barley malt, mixing until creamy. Add to cereal and stir. Simmer another 20 to 30 minutes until cereal is soft and cooked. Make sure heat is low and pan is covered with lid, or cereal will burn.

Serves 3

Nutritive values per serving:	CAL	PRO (gm)	FAT (gm)	CHO (gm)
	207	5	0	47

Awesome Apple Pudding

$1\frac{1}{2}$ cups whole wheat flour
2 cups skim milk
$\frac{1}{4}$ cup undiluted frozen apple juice, thawed
2 teaspoons vanilla extract
4 egg whites
4 apples, peeled and sliced
$\frac{1}{4}$ cup orange juice
1 teaspoon ground cinnamon
Dash ground ginger

Combine flour, milk, apple juice concentrate, and vanilla in a bowl. Beat egg whites until frothy, add to flour mixture, and mix well. Arrange the peeled apple slices in a layer on the bottom of a medium nonstick baking dish. Sprinkle orange juice and half the ground cinnamon over the apples. Add dash of ground ginger and other half of ground cinnamon to the batter. Pour the batter over the apples and bake in a 400°F oven for 30 minutes. Cut the pudding into squares and serve.

Serves 4

Nutritive values per serving:

195

CAL	PRO (gm)	FAT (gm)	CHO (gm)
374	12.2	1.6	78

Super Potato Salad

2 pounds red potatoes
½ cup chopped celery
½ cup finely chopped bell pepper
1 large onion, chopped coarse
3 hard-boiled eggs, chopped, with yolks removed
1 clove garlic, minced fine
½ cup uncreamed, low-fat cottage cheese
⅓ cup skim milk
⅛ teaspoon dry mustard
¼ teaspoon celery seed
¼ teaspoon dried dill
1 tablespoon vinegar
1 tablespoon fresh lemon juice
½ pound fresh shrimp, peeled, deveined, and chopped coarse
   Fresh coarsely ground white pepper

Boil potatoes until tender, about 25 to 28 minutes. Cube potatoes and mix in bowl with celery, green pepper, onion, and eggs. Beat together garlic, cheese, milk, spices, vinegar, and lemon juice. Combine dressing with potatoes, adding shrimp. Chill before serving. Add pepper and serve.

Serves 8

Nutritive values per serving:

CAL	PRO (gm)	FAT (gm)	CHO (gm)
130	11	2	19

Linguine and Clam Sauce

15 ounces Basic Marinara Sauce (see index)
½ cup chopped clams
½ large green pepper, chopped
2 tablespoons chopped garlic
1 onion, chopped fine
½ teaspoon freshly ground pepper
   Dash hot red pepper flakes, crushed
8 ounces linguine
   Water

Pour sauce into a pot and add clams, green pepper, garlic, onion, pepper, and crushed red pepper. Simmer for 30 minutes on very low flame. Drop linguine into 3 quarts of boiling water and boil until done to taste. Drain linguine and serve with clam sauce poured on top.

Serves 4

Nutritive values per serving:

	CAL	PRO (gm)	FAT (gm)	CHO (gm)
	278	21.3	2.2	69

Vegetables and Rice

1 cup raw brown rice
1 cup pineapple juice
1 cup fresh grapefruit juice
½ cup chopped onion
½ cup chopped celery
¼ cup chopped green pepper
1 teaspoon chopped fresh parsley
½ teaspoon chili powder
⅛ teaspoon freshly ground pepper

Put raw brown rice in a nonstick skillet and heat. Add pineapple juice, grapefruit juice, onion, celery, green pepper, parsley, chili powder, and pepper and mix well. Simmer, covered, for 40 minutes or until done.

Serves 4

Nutritive values per serving:

	CAL	PRO (gm)	FAT (gm)	CHO (gm)
	254	5	1	56.7

Brown Rice and Kidney Beans

1 cup brown rice
½ medium-sized onion, chopped
1 tablespoon whole wheat flour
2 tablespoons water
1 cup water
1 15-ounce can red kidney beans, rinsed 3 times to remove salt
1 tablespoon chopped fresh parsley
¼ teaspoon chili powder
¼ teaspoon minced garlic
⅛ teaspoon freshly ground pepper
Dash red hot pepper sauce

Cook rice according to directions on package. In a nonstick frying pan, fry onions until slightly brown. Mix flour with 2 tablespoons water and blend mixture into fried onions. Cook for 3 minutes and add 1 cup water. Cook until slightly thickened and add beans and seasonings. Add rice, mix well, and serve.

Serves 4

Nutritive values per serving:

	CAL	PRO (gm)	FAT (gm)	CHO (gm)
	302	11.4	1.4	61

Banana Orange Shake

1 cup orange juice
1 banana
2 ice cubes
½ cup low-fat yogurt
Dash ground cinnamon
Sprig fresh mint

Combine all ingredients except mint in a blender on medium speed until smooth and fluffy. Top with sprig of fresh mint and serve.

Serves 1

Nutritive values per serving:

	CAL	PRO (gm)	FAT (gm)	CHO (gm)
	311	9.2	59.4	2.5

Chicken Gumbo

1 16-ounce can okra, drained
¼ cup chopped onion
¼ large green pepper, chopped
4 cups chicken broth
4 tomatoes
½ teaspoon freshly ground pepper
1 cup diced cooked chicken
1 bay leaf
1 tablespoon chopped fresh parsley
3 cups cooked rice

In a nonstick pan, cook okra, onion, and green pepper on low heat until onion is soft. Stir in chicken broth, tomatoes, pepper, chicken, bay leaf, and parsley. Simmer, uncovered, for 20 minutes. Serve with ¾ cup rice per bowl.

Serves 4

Nutritive values per serving:

CAL	PRO (gm)	FAT (gm)	CHO (gm)
285	15	2	54

REFERENCES

Aberg, B. L., Ekman, R. & Falk, U. et al. *Arch Environ Health*, 1969, *19*, 478.

American Medical Association, Council on Foods and Nutrition, *Nutrients in Processed Foods*, Acton, Mass: Publishing Science Group, 1974.

Anderson, B. B., Perry, G. M., Modell, G. B. et al, *Br J Haematol*, 1979, *41*, 497.

Anderson, G. et al, *Diabetes*, 1982, *31*, 212

Bailey, D. A. et al, *Am J Clin Nutr*, 1970, *23*, 905.

Baker, S. J. & De Maeyer, E. M., *Am J Clin Nutr*, 1979, *32*, 368.

Bantle, J. P. et al, *N Engl J Med*, 1983, *309*, 7.

Bergstrom, J., Hermansen, I., Hultman, E., et al. *Acta Physiol Scand.*, 1967, *71*, 140.

Bistrian, B. R. et al, *JAMA*, 1974, *320*, 858.

Bistrian, B. R. et al, *JAMA*, 1976, *325*, 1567.

Bollet, A. J., & Owens, S. *Am J Clin Nutr*, 1973, *23*, 931.

Bonen, A. et al, *J Appl Physiol*, 1981, *50*, 766.

Bradley, R. L. & Hugunin, A. G. *Safety of Foods*, 1980, 350.

Butterworth, C. E., Santini, J. R. & Frommeyer, W. B., *J. Clin Invest*, 1963, *42*, 1929.

Butterworth, C. E., *Nutrition Today*, 1974, *9*, 4.

Calloway, D. H., *Nutrition Reviews*, 1962, *20*, 257.

Calloway, D. H., et al. *J Nutrition*, 1971, *101*, 775.

Camarini-Davalos, R. A., Hanover, R. (Eds) *Treatment of Early Diabetes*, Advances in Experimental Medicine and Biology Vol 119, New York: Plenum 1979.

Clement, D. et al, *Canadian Med Assoc J.*, 1977, *177*, 614.

Clements, J. E., Anderson, B. B., *Biochem Biophys Acts*, 1980, *362*, 159.

Cohen, A. M. et al, Effect of interchanging bread and sucrose as main source of carbohydrate in low fat diet on glucose tolerance curve of healthy volunteer subject. *Am J Clin Nutr*, 1966, *19*, 59.

Colgan, M., Effects of vitamin and mineral supplementation on physiology and performance of athletes. Paper presented at the Rockefeller University, New York, March 1981. (a)

Colgan, M., *Science*, 1981, *214*, 744 (b).

Colgan, M., *Your Personal Vitamin Profile*, New York: Morrow, 1982.

Colgan, M., Effects of nutrient supplements on athletic performance, paper presented to the U.S. Navy Research and Development Center, April 1983. Carlsbad CA, Colgan Institute Publication, 1983 (a).

Colgan, M., *Copper contamination of drinking water in Upper East Side Manhattan*, Carlsbad, CA: Colgan Institute Publications, 1983 (b).

Colgan, M. & Colgan, L., *Nutrition and Health*, 1984, *3*, 1.

Colgan, M., *Optimum Nutrition for Athletes*, London: Mueller *in press*, publication, Spring 1985.

Consolazio, F. C., et al, *J Nutr*, 1963, *79*, 407.

Consolazio, F. C., et al (Eds), *Physiological Measurements of Metabolic Functions in Man*, New York: McGraw-Hill, 1963.

Consolazio, F. C., et al. *Nutrition Report Int*, 1975, *11*, 231.

Consumer Reports, 1981, July, 376.

Costill, D. L., Kammer, W. F. & Fisher, A., *Arch Environ Health*, 1970, *21*, 520.

Costill, D. L., et al, *J Appl Physiol*, 1977, *43*, 695.

Costill, D. L. *A Scientific Approach to Distance Running*, Los Altos, California: Track & Field News, 1979.

Costill, D. L. & Miller, J. M., *Int J Sports Med*, 1980, *1*, 2.

Costill, D. L. et al *Am J. Clin Nutr*, 1981, *34*, 1831.

Costill, D. L., in Haskel, W., et al (Eds), *Nutrition and Athletic Performance*, Palo Alto, CA: Bull Publishing, 1982, 16.

Crapo, P. A., et al, *Am J Clin Nutr*, 1981, *34*, 184.

Crapper, D. R., et al, *Brain*, 1976, *99*, 67.

Dohm, G. L., et al *J Appl Physiol*, 1982, *53*, 27.

Dressendorfer, R. H., et al, *JAMA*, 1981, *246*, 1215.

Edington, D. E., *The Biology of Physical Activity*, London: Houghton Mifflin, 1976, Ch 14.

Ehn, L., Carlmark, B. & Hoglund, S., *Med Sci Spors*, 1980, *12*, 61.

Emmerson, B. T., *Ann Rheum Dis*, 1974, *33*, 276.

Evans, W. J., et al. *Physician & Sports Med*, 1983, *11*, 63.

Fairbanks, V. F., et al (Eds), *Clinical Disorders of Iron Metabolism*, New York: Grune and Stratton, 1971.

Fink, W., in Haskell, W. (Ed) *Nutrition and Athletic Performance*, Palo Alto CA: Bull Publishing 1982, 52.

Food and Nutrition Board, *Folic Acid*, Washington DC: National Academy of Sciences, 1977.

Forun, B., et al *Am J Clin Nutr*, 1977, *30*, 1983.

Foster, C., et al, *Med Sci Sports*, 1979, *11*, 1.

Frederickson, L. A., et al, *Med Sci Sports*, 1983, *15*, 271.

Ganther, H. E., Levander, O. A. & Cheng, L., *Micronutrient Interactions*, New York: New York Academy of Sciences, 1980, 212.

Garza, C., Scrimshaw, N. S., Young, V. R. *J Nutrition*, 1977, *107*, 335.

Gliesman, E. & Mertz, W., *Metab*, 1966, *15*, 510.

Gontzea, I., et al, *Nutrition Reports Int*, 1974, *10*, 35.

Greenleaf, J. E., Olsson, K. & Saltin, B., *Acta Physiol Scand*, 1969, *330*, Suppl.

Greenleaf, J. E., in Haskell, W., et all (Eds) *Nutrition & Athletic Performance* Palo Alto CA: Bull Publishing 1982, 34.

Grey, G. O., et al, *JAMA*, 1970, *211*, 105.

Hanes, I., *First Health and Nutrition Examination Survey, United States*, 1971–72 DHEW Publication 76-1219-1, Rockville, MD: DHEW 1976.

Harris, R. S. & Levenberg, R. K., in Harris, R. S. & Von Loesecke, H. (Eds) *Nutritional Evaluation of Food Processing*, Westport, Conn: Avi Publishing, 1960, 47.

Harris, R. S. & Von Loesecke, H. (eds) *Nutritional Evaluation of Food Processing*, Westport, Conn: Avi Publishing, 1960, 47.

Harris, R. S. & Karmas, E., (Eds) *Nutritional Evaluation of Food Processing*, Westport, Conn: Avi Publishing, 1975.

Hegsted, D. M., *Federation Proceedings*, 1963, *22*, 1424.

Herbert, V., *Trans Assoc Am Physicians*, 1962, *75*, 307.

Herbert, V., *Am J Clin Nutr*, 1968, *21*, 743.

Herbert, V., *New England J Med*, 1971, *284*, 976.

Herbert, V., *Seminars in Nuclear Medicine*, 1972, *2*, 220.

Howald, H., et al, *Ann NY Acad Sci*, 1975, *258*, 458.

Inoue, G., Fujita, Y., Niiyama, Y. *J Nutrition*, 1973, *103*, 1673.

Jenkins, D. J., Wolever, T. M., Taylor, R. H. et al *Am J Clin Nutr*, 1981, *34*, 184.

Keller, K. & Schwarzkopf, R., *Physician and Sports Med*, 1984, *12*, 89.

Kelsay, J. L., et al, The effect of kind of carbohydrate in the diet and use of oral contraceptives on metabolism of young women. I. Blood and urinary lactate, uric acid and phosphorus, *Am J Clin Nutr*, 1977, *30*, 2016.
Klevay, L. M., et al, *JAMA*, 1979, *241*, 1916.
Klevay, L. M., in Levander, O. A. & Cheng, L., (Eds), *Micronutrient Interactions*, New York: New York Academy of Sciences, 1980, 140.
Kolata, G., *Science*, 1984, *223*, 381.
Krichevsky, D., Davidson, L. M. & Shapiro, I. L., *Am J Clin Nutr*, 1980, *33*, 1869.
Krochta, J. M. & Feinberg, B., in Harris, R. S. & Karmas, E., (Eds), *Nutritional Evaluation of Food Processing*, Westport Conn: Avi Publishing, 1975, 98.
Lavoie, A., et al, *Clin Sci Mol Med*, 1974, *47*, 617.
Levander, O. A., in Levander, O. A. & Cheng, L. (Eds), *Micronutrient Interactions*, New York: New York Academy of Sciences, 1980, 227.
Levander, O. A. & Cheng, L, (Eds), *Micronutrient Interactions*, New York: New York Academy of Sciences, 1980, 140.
Levene, L., Evans, W. J. et al, *J Appl Physiol*, 1983, *55*, 1767.
Liu, A., & Morris, C., *Am J Clin Nutr*, 1978, *31*, 972.
Linkswiler, H. M., Joyce, C. L. & Anand, C. R., *New York Acad Sciences Trans*, 1974, *36*, 333.
Locksley, R., *West J Med*, 1980, *133*, 493.
Lund, D. B., in Harris, R. S. & Karmas, E., (Eds) *Nutritional Evaluation of Food Processing*, Westport Conn: Avi Publishing, 1975, 205.
Machlin, J., Gabriel, E., in Levander, O. A. & Cheng, L. (Eds) *Micronutrient Interactions*, New York: New York Academy of Sciences, 1980, 98.
Mahaffey, K. R., Rader, J. I., in Levander, O. A. & Cheng, L. (Eds) *Micronutrient Interactions*, New York: New York Academy of Sciences, 1980, 285.
Margaria, R., (Ed) *Exercise at Altitude*, Amsterdam: Exerpta Media, 1967.
Marks, J., *Vitamins in Health and Disease*, London: Churchill, 1968.
Mason, K. E., Young, J. O., in Muth, O. H. (Ed) *Selenium in Biomedicine*., Westport, Conn: Avi Publishing, 1967.
Mertz, W., in Shapcott, D., Hubert, J. (Eds), Chromium in Nutrition and Metabolism, Amsterdam: Elsevier North Holland, 1979, 1.
Mimson, P. L., et al (Eds), *Vitamins and Hormones*, Vol 34, New York: Academic Press, 1976.
Mitchell, D. G., Aldous, K. M., *Environ Health Perspect*, 1974, *7*, 59.
Moroff, S. V., Bass, D. E., *J Appl Physiol*, 1965, *20*, 267.
National Academy of Sciences, *Reports of the Subcommittee on the Geochemical Environment in Relation to Health and Disease*. Washington DC: National Academy of Sciences, 1974–1978.
National Research Council, *Toward Healthful Diets*, Washington DC: National Academy of Sciences, 1980.
Nationwide Food Consumption Survey 1977–1978, Prelim Report No 2 Washington DC: USDA, 1980.
Nielsen, F. H., Hunt, C. D., Uthus, E. O., in Levander, O. E. & Cheng, L. (Eds) *Micronutrient Interactions*, New York: New York Academy of Sciences 1980, 152.
Norman, A. W., (Ed), *Vitamin D: Biochemical, Chemical and Clinical Aspects Related to Calcium Metabolism*, Berlin: Walter De Gruyter, 1977.
Norman, A. W. (Ed), *Vitamin D: Basic Research and Its Clinical Applications*, Berlin: Walter De Gruyter 1979.
Norms for hair concentrations of Cu, Ni, Cd, Hg, Pb, in subjects who avoid sources of metal contamination of food, water and air. Colgan Institute of Nutritional Science, Carlsbad, CA, 1983.
Ondreicka, R., Kortus, J., Ginter, E. in Skoryna, S. C. and Waldron-Edward, D. (Eds) *Intestinal Incorporation of Metal Ions, Trace Elements and Radionuclides*, Oxford: Pergamon 1971, 293.
Painter, N., *Ann Royal Coll Surg Eng.* 1964, *34*, 98.
Parr, R. B., Bachman, L. A., Moss, R. A., *Physician and Sports Med*, 1984, *4*, 81.
Patrias, B., Olson, O., *J Agriculture and Food Chemistry* 1967, *15*, 448.
Paul, A. A., Southgate, D. A., *Composition of Foods 4th Edition*, Oxford: Elsevier/North-Holland, 1978.
Philips, M., Baetz, A. (Eds), *Diets and Resistance to Disease: Advances in Experimental Medicine and Biology, Vol 35*, New York: Plenum 1981.
Recommended Dietary Allowances: Ninth Revised Addition, Washington DC: National Academy of Sciences 1980.
Reiser, S., et al, Isocaloric exchange of dietary starch and sucrose in humans. II. Effect on fasting blood insulin, glucose, and glycogen and on insulin and glucose response to a sucrose load, *Am J Clin Nutr*, 1979, *32*, 2206.
Reiser, S. in Bland, G., (Ed) *Medical Aspects of Clinical Nutrition*, New Canaan, Conn., 1983, 133.
Rennie, M. J., et al. *Biochemistry Soc Trans*, 1980, *8*, 499.
Riales, P., Albrink, R., *Am J Clin Nutr*, 1981, *34*, 2670.
Rodriguez, M. S., *J Nutr*, 1978, *108*, 1983.
Royal College of Physicians, *Medical Aspects of Dietary Fiber*, London: Pitman, 1980.
Sable, H. Z., Gubler, C. J., (Eds), *Thiamin: Twenty Years of Progress*, New York: New York Academy of Sciences, 1982.
Sauberlich, H. E., in Levander, O. A. & Cheng, L., (Eds), *Micronutrient Interactions*, New York: New York Academy of Sciences 1980, 80.
Schroeder, H. A. *Am J Clin Nutr*, 1971, *24*, 562.
Shils, M., in Levander, O. A. & Cheng, L. (Eds), *Micronutrient Interactions*, New York: New York Academy of Sciences 1980, 165.
Solyst, J. T. et al, Effect of dietary sucrose in humans on blood uric acid, phosphorus, fructose, and lactic acid responses to a sucrose load, *Nutr Metabol*, 1980, *24*, 182.
Spencer, H., et al, in Levander, O. A. & Cheng, L., *Micronutrient Interactions*, New York: New York Academy of Sciences 1980, 181.
Spiller, G. A., Kay, R. P. (Eds), *Medical Aspects of Dietary Fiber*, New York: Plenum 1980.
Spivey, M. R., et al, in Levander, O. A. & Cheng, L., *Micronutrient Interactions*, New York: New York Academy of Sciences, 1980, 249.
Stoewsand, G. S. in Graham H. D. (Ed) *The Safety of Foods* Westport Conn: Avi Publishing, 1980, *423*.
Sturgeon, P., Shoden, A., *Am J Clin Nutr*, 1975, *24*, 469.
Ten State Nutritional Survey, DHEW Publications 72-8130 No.s 1, 2, and 3, Rockville, MD: DHEW 1972.
The Surgeon General, *Healthy People*, DHEW Publications No.s 79-55071 and 79-55071 A Washington DC : Govt Printing Office, 1979, Trowell, H.C., Burkitt, D. P. (Eds), *Western Diseases: Their Emergence and Prevention*, Cambridge, Mass: Harvard University Press, 1981.
Tzagournis, M., *Am J Clin Nutr*, 1978, *31*, 1437.
Underwood, E. J., *Trace Elements in Human and Animal Nutrition 4th Edition*, New York: Academic Press 1977.
USDA, *National Food Situation*, USDA Circ 150, Washington DC: USDA, 1974.
Vander, A. J. *Nutrition, Stress & Toxic Chemicals*, Ann Arbor: University of Michigan Press, 1981, Ch 4.
Veller, O., *Scandi Clin Invest*, 1968, *21*, 157.
Visagie, M. E., DuPlessis, J. P., Laubscher, N. F., Effects of Vitamin C supplementation of black mine workers, *S African Med J*, 1975, *9*, 889–892.
Watt, B. K., & Merrill, A. L., *Composition of Foods*, Washington DC: USDA, 1963.
Weinsier, R. L., et al, *Am J Clin Nutr*, 1979, *32*, 418.
Williams, M. H., In Haskell, W. L., et al (Eds) *Nutrition and Athletic Performances*, Palo Alto, CA: Bull Publishing 1981, 106.
Williams, R. J., et al, *Lancet, 1950, 1*, 287.
Williams, R., *Biochemical Individuality*, New York: Wiley, 1956.
Williams, R. J., Deason, ., *Proc Nat Acad Sci USA*, 1967, *57*, 1638.
Williams, R. J., Heffley, J. D., Yew M. *Perspect Bio Med*, 1973, *17*, 1.

200

INDEX

203